HANDBOOK OF INTERPROFESSIONAL PRACTICE

A Guide for Interprofessional Education & Collaborative Care

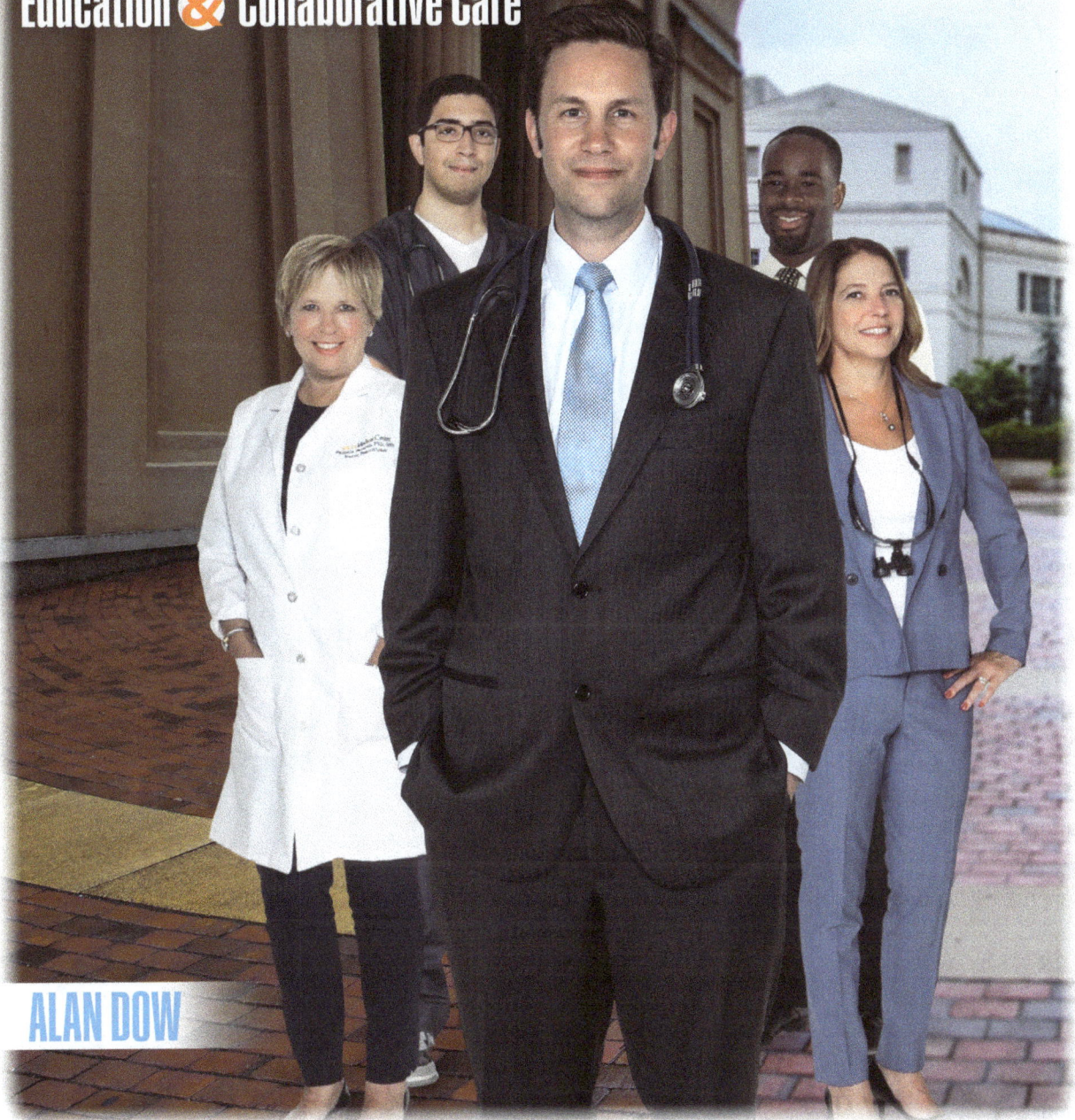

ALAN DOW

Kendall Hunt
publishing company

Photo used with permission of Virginia Commonwealth University.

Kendall Hunt
publishing company

www.kendallhunt.com
Send all inquiries to:
4050 Westmark Drive
Dubuque, IA 52004-1840

Contents

Acknowledgments

First and foremost, I need to thank all of the patients who have made me a better collaborator. While healthcare is challenging work, our patients face the biggest challenges. Their strength and perseverance inspire me, especially when their resolve cracks enough so that their frustration or grief spills through momentarily. We often wish we could do more than possible, and, because of them, sometimes we do.

My colleagues also deserve much of the credit for my journey. I have been fortunate to have wonderful partners in this work, both in Richmond and elsewhere. We are usually learning, and regularly laughing, both of which I consider to be marks of success. In this group, I also include my students, who are always teaching me something; they continue to amaze me as their lives take flight.

I owe specific, profound gratitude to Sheldon Retchin and George Thibault who provided me the opportunity to do this work.

My only sadness about writing this book was that my friend and admired colleague, Scott Reeves, never had a chance to provide his undoubtedly insightful critique. Rest in peace, Scott.

Thanks also to the group at Kendall Hunt Publishing, specifically Curtis Ross, with his relentless enthusiasm, and Bev Kraus, who worked miracles around my deadlines. And thanks to Kristin Walinski and Sandy Hausrath at Scribe for their help with editing this book and making it so much better.

Finally, my greatest collaborators are, as ever, my family, especially Tara, Sylvia, and Ezra. It turns out that being an international expert in healthcare collaboration doesn't mean you actually know what you're doing. When I get caught up in the tumult of life, they show me the path forward. I'm not perfect, but I'm always trying to get better.

SECTION 1

Interprofessional Practice and This Book

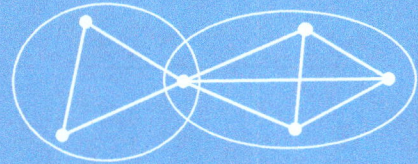

CHAPTER 1

Introduction to the Handbook for Interprofessional Practice

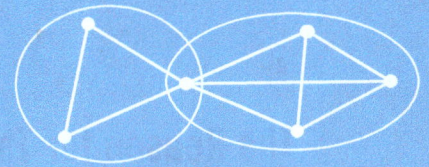

The purpose of this chapter is to orient you to the field of interprofessional practice, the reason for this book, and its overall structure. Each chapter starts with a brief summary paragraph as well as some objectives. The initial summary paragraph will give you an overview of the chapter and the learning objectives for each chapter. By the end of this chapter, you will be able to:

▸ identify the importance of better interprofessional practice,

▸ define terminology related to interprofessional practice and how this terminology is used in the context of this book, and

▸ describe the structure of this book.

Initial Reflection Questions

Throughout the book, you will be presented questions to support your learning and sidebar that either expand on a point or provide supplementary information. Read more about initial reflection questions in this sidebar.

This book is about *interprofessional practice*. Simply defined, interprofessional practice is when people from different professions collaborate to improve the health of patients and communities. Yet, while this definition is simple, interprofessional practice can get challenging very quickly. Consider these questions:

■ What are the problems that we hope to solve through better interprofessional practice? Why haven't we already solved these problems? What barriers are there to solving these problems?

> **The Importance of Reflection**
> At the start of each chapter, you'll find some initial reflection questions. The purpose of these questions is to get you thinking about the topic. It turns out thinking about questions like this makes what you learn stick in your brain better. Take a moment to think about the answers and consider using the white space below each question to jot down some thoughts. If you are using this book as part of a class, these questions might also be part of an assignment.

- What prevents us from having optimal interprofessional practice? Compared to the problems that you noted above, are these barriers to optimal interprofessional practice and to solving these problems the same or different?

The Reason for This Book

This book strives to help you work better within the healthcare system. The healthcare system is described as a complex system. A complex system has lots of parts, and these parts can interact in many different ways.

Think of all the parts of the healthcare system: patients, practitioners, medications, procedures, tests, buildings, technology, and many more. All of these parts could interact in any number of ways to help a patient. Your job is to be a part of this complex system that helps your patients achieve the best health outcomes.

Fortunately, you are smart, well-trained, and committed to your patients. However, the challenges ahead of you can be daunting. This handbook seeks to be your guide as you navigate this complex system and provide the best possible care for your patients.

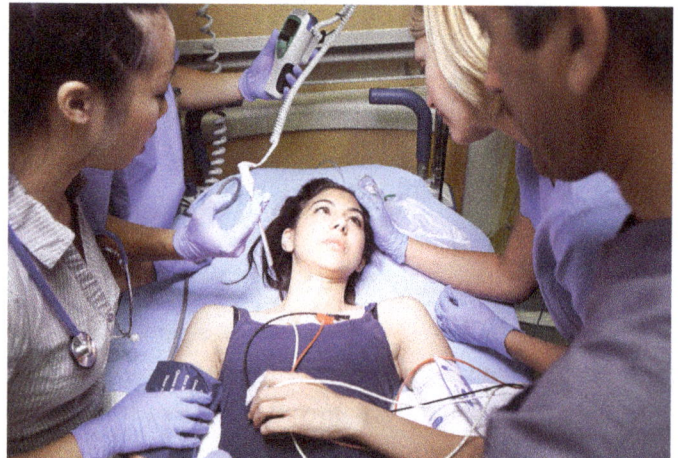

© Monkey Business Images/Shutterstock.com

Let's talk about some of these challenges. Patients present with lots of different needs, such as making a diagnosis, promoting healthy behaviors, educating about ongoing problems and therapies, or screening for unknown problems. Some of these needs—like having an appendectomy—require care in hospitals. When most of us think about health, we think about situations like that.

But it turns out that typical healthcare only accounts for about 10 percent of the variation in people's health (Figure 1.1). While most of us work or will work in typical healthcare settings like hospitals, clinics, and rehabilitation settings, it's critical to recognize that, while most of what goes on in these facilities is important, it does not address the underlying causes of poor health outcomes. Health depends much more on socioeconomic factors, individual behaviors, genetics, and the environment.

Think about smoking—it's still the biggest preventable cause of disease. And it's mainly a behavior that occurs outside of typical healthcare. It's the product of peer groups, advertising, untreated psychological disease, and other social determinants of health. And, whether you get emphysema or other downstream effects also depends on your genetics and on how much secondhand smoke you are exposed to.

We're facing huge barriers to decreasing the health effects of smoking. And, we're making progress. Over the past several decades, smoking rates are down, and so are the health impacts. Now the question is, what can you and I do to build on this progress?

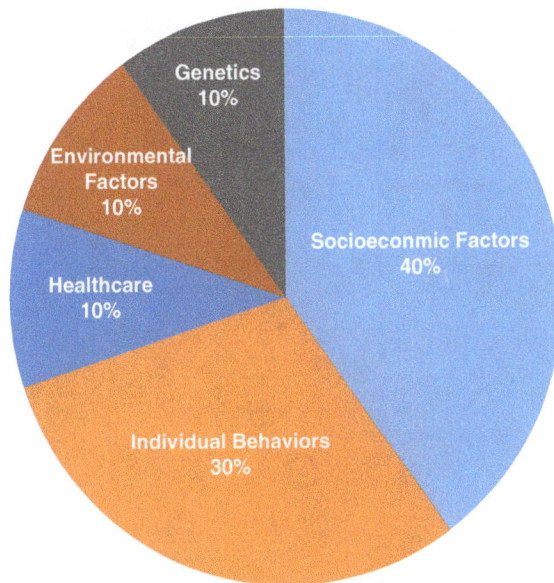

Figure 1.1 The Determinants of Health. Source: Alan Dow based on data from Schroeder SA. NEJM. 2007.

As we go through this book, I want you to think about questions like this. My goal is to have you think broadly about health and not just focus on the healthcare system as it exists today. We're really good at what we currently do, and our biggest health challenges happen beyond the capacity of our current systems for care. If your job is to improve the health of your patients, think about how you can have the most beneficial impact on society and all the determinants of health.

This is not to say that we have perfect systems in typical healthcare settings. We know that at least 100,000 and possibly as many 400,000 people in the United States die each year from consequences of medical errors. In fact, these startling statistics drove the initial emphasis on interprofessional practice. In about 70 percent of these medical errors, failures of interprofessional practice, such as lapses in communication, are a contributing cause. Anyone who has been a patient or had a family member as a patient can probably relate a tale of some sort of miscommunication in healthcare. While our goal is to help people, the complex and high-stakes nature of healthcare means that we sometimes do the opposite. Better interprofessional practice is part of the solution to these safety challenges.

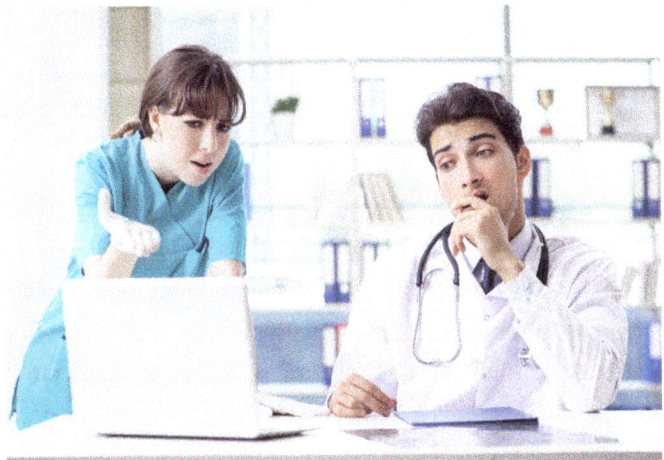

It's also important to keep health equity in mind. For example, in my city, two children who grow up five miles apart have a 20-year gap in life expectancy (Figure 1.1). Most cities have similar disparities. The biggest predictor of this gap in the United States is race. While every country has a different history, in the United States, our past racial inequities drive our current health inequities. You alone can't solve this problem, but you and your colleagues can work to address it.

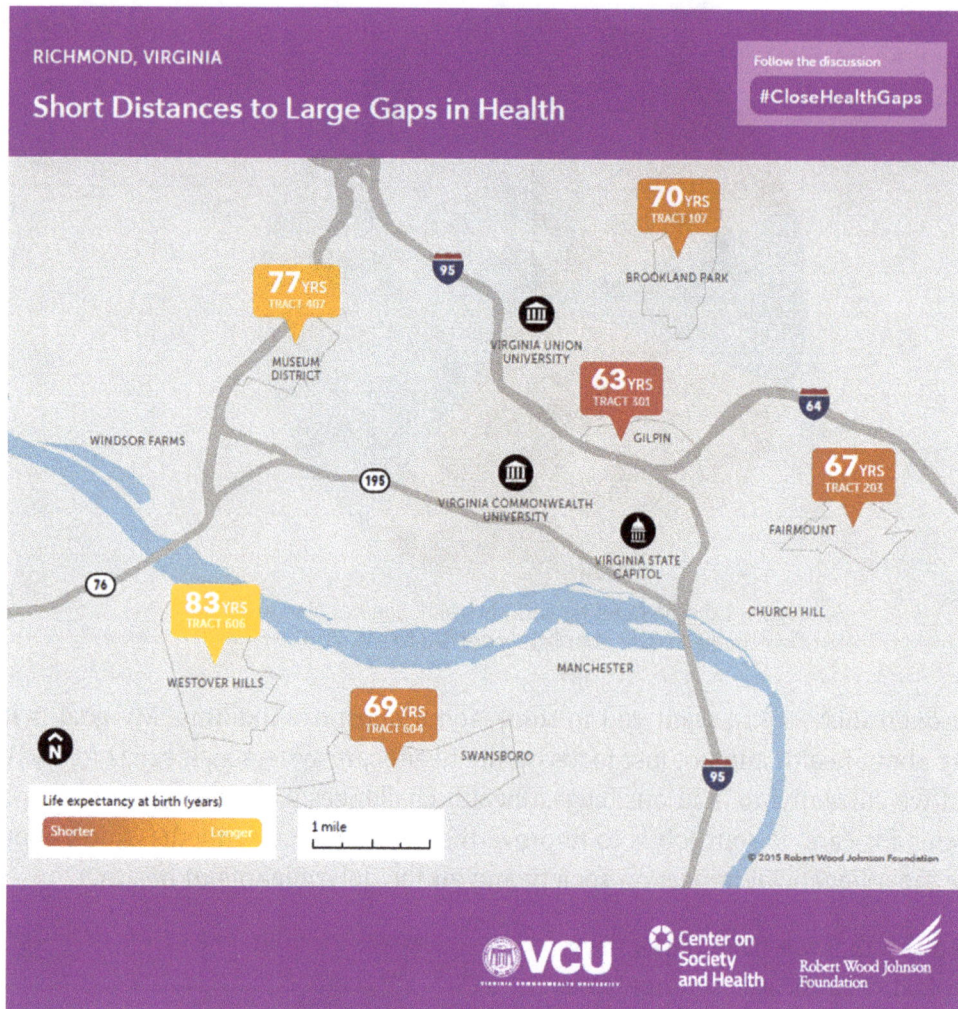

Figure 1.2 The Effect of 5 Miles on Life Expectancy. Source: Reprinted with permission from the VCU Center on Society and Health.

Race is not the only factor that influences health equity. Income level is also correlated with health and may become an even bigger health predictor than race over the next few decades in the United States. And there are differences in health outcomes correlated with gender, ethnicity, sexual orientation, and many other factors. This book is not going to tell you how to fix these deep-seated societal problems. But I want you to have this context and think about how broader societal factors shape the health of your patients. You might end up making a greater difference in society with work beyond typical healthcare settings. And interprofessional collaboration will be essential.

We are also at an important moment in the history of our world. Because of immunizations, decreased violence, and better healthcare, we are all living longer. People are also having fewer children than ever before. As a result, the percentage of the global population that is 65 years old or older will increase from about 8 percent today to over 16 percent in 2050 (Figure 1.3). As people age, they develop more chronic diseases like hypertension and diabetes and need more health services. Meanwhile, the percentage of children under five is decreasing and is predicted to drop from about 9 percent today to about 7 percent in 2050. These children are our future health workforce, and their numbers are shrinking. We may have twice as much need for health services in the future with 25 percent fewer people to provide these services.

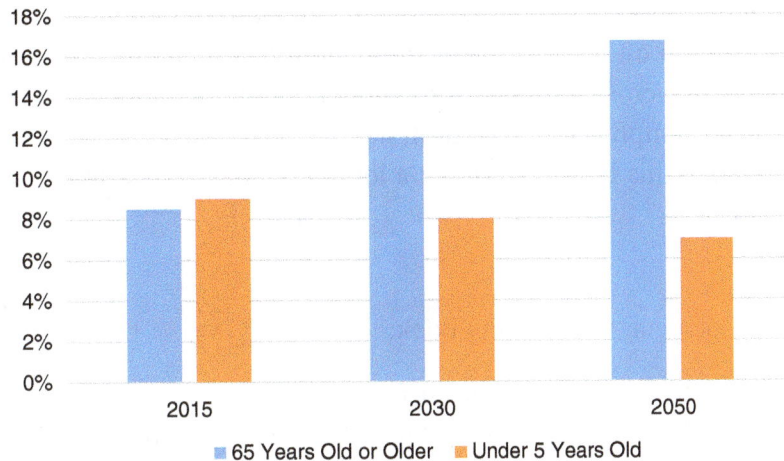

Figure 1.3 Global Population by Age. Source: Alan Dow based on data from the U.S. Census Bureau.

Think about a typical baby boomer over the age of 65. We know from studies that these people often have two or more chronic health conditions. As people add health conditions, their health needs multiply: prescribing medication can be more complex because of interactions between drugs and disease, counseling has to be tailored to all health conditions, and choosing the best path forward becomes less easily defined by evidence as it has to become more individualized. The point is that we will have to figure out how to provide more care with fewer healthcare practitioners. And if you add in the fact that health services are already a large percentage of many governments' budgets, being efficient while keeping people healthy will become even more of an imperative.

So, there are a lot of challenges before us: medical errors, health inequities, an aging population, and the high cost of healthcare. But, overall, we are a healthier and more prosperous planet than we have ever been. I am optimistic that we will overcome these challenges for one big reason—you and your peers. Which brings us back to the focus of this book: interprofessional practice.

Interprofessional practice is defined as when individuals from two or more healthcare professions work together to improve health outcomes. Traditionally, healthcare professions have not collaborated as well as they might have. Here are a few of the barriers to collaboration in healthcare:

- practitioners are educated separately;
- workspaces are divided into separate territories like the nurses' stations, the physician workroom, and the pharmacy;
- professional cultures develop in opposition to one another, and this conflict is reinforced by battles around licensing and professional responsibilities; and
- healthcare occurs in clinics and hospitals while the people we serve would prefer to spend most of their time elsewhere.

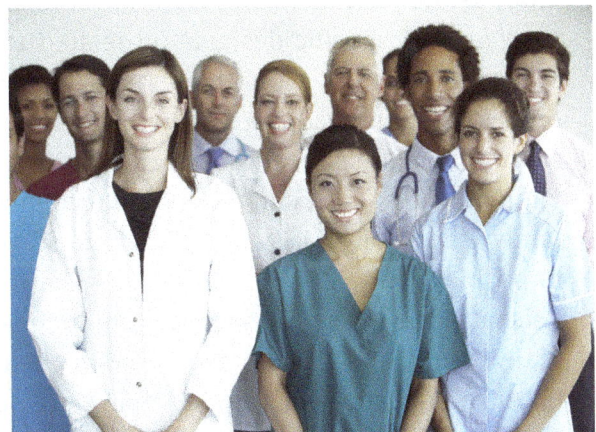

We could spend a lot of time on the barriers to collaboration and the underlying reasons it doesn't happen, and we will touch on many of these throughout this book, but, for now, recognize that we have failed to collaborate across professions to support health as much as we could have. That failure has led to a renewed emphasis on interprofessional practice across the globe and has brought us together in the context of this book. We've got a lot to do. Let's get started.

Terminology

Some notes on terminology as we start the book:

- As I have been doing, I will use the term *interprofessional practice* to define collaboration in healthcare among different professions. Other terms have been used elsewhere; for example, the World Health Organization uses the term "interprofessional collaborative practice," while others use the term "interprofessional care." To keep it simple, I will stick with interprofessional practice.
- *Interprofessional education* is training that seeks to improve interprofessional practice.
- When we talk about a collection of healthcare professions, I will refer to them as a *group*. Others have used the term "team," but "team" has a specific meaning, and "group" is a more general term to describe how healthcare professionals interact in most settings. We will dive much more deeply into this issue in chapter 4.
- I also differentiate between healthcare practitioners, healthcare providers, and healthcare workers. A *healthcare practitioner* is a trained member of the healthcare workforce. Typically, he or she has a license and works directly with individuals with health needs. This group is the main audience for this book, and this term is the one I use the most. A *healthcare provider* is a specific designation related to billing for health services (at least in the United States). I generally avoid this term. A *healthcare worker* is the broadest term; it includes anyone working in healthcare, including healthcare practitioners and also groups such as clerical staff, custodial service workers, and administrators. All of these groups are essential for providing the best care, and we should recognize and support their contributions. They could certainly learn from this book, though most examples will be focused on providing care directly to people.
- I also use the term *healthcare system* to mean all the pieces that fit together to support health. Many argue, and I agree, that we don't really have a healthcare system in the United States because our pieces to support health are so fragmented. That fragmentation is actually part of the reason for this book. But even if our healthcare system is lousy, most of the pieces are there, and our job is to fit them together as best we can for our patients. In addition, by healthcare system, I do not mean a specific hospital system but rather all the different entities that may serve a community. Consider this broadly: a small, nonprofit clinic focused partially on supporting health is as much a part of the healthcare system as a multibillion-dollar hospital.
- *Health services* is the term I use for all activities that support health. These activities have a wide range, from health education in a school to brain surgery in an academic medical center. Sometimes, the border between health services and non-health services is blurry. Are good

sanitation, clean water, and nutritious food choices health services? I don't think that question has a clear answer, but my inclination is for us to think broadly about health and health services.

- Finally, I will generally refer to people who receive health services as *patients*. But when does someone become a patient or stop being a patient? Certainly, when someone is admitted to a hospital, "patient" seems like the right term. But what about after that person is discharged? What if you see that person in passing at the grocery store—is he or she still a patient? Being a patient is just a role that an individual might assume, like being a mother, a student, a supervisor, or a backup singer. It's only a part of who someone is. That being said, for the most part, I will use the term *patient* for lack of a less cumbersome term. Occasionally, I will also refer to *community members* to mean people who might receive health services away from typical locations for health services like clinics or hospitals.And I should note that wherever I use "patients," we could substitute "patients and their families." Health is certainly not something we pursue alone, especially as children or older adults.

The Structure of This Book

Being a book, this work is made up of a sequence of chapters, yet interprofessional practice is not a linear arena. I have tried to put the chapters in a logical order, but you may find that you want to skip ahead and then jump back depending on your particular inclination. Often, I will refer you ahead or back to another chapter if a topic is covered in greater depth elsewhere. Here is an overview of the remaining chapters so you know what's to come.

Chapters 2 and 3 focus on individual team members. Chapter 2 discusses the concept of *scope of practice* and how licensure and regulations shape healthcare professions. Chapter 3 then talks about how different professions take on different *roles and responsibilities* in their daily work based on factors in the practice setting. Here, I hope to have you think about your own professional identity and how it relates to and evolves with the professional identity of other healthcare practitioners.

Chapters 4 through 8 look at how groups of practitioners work in the healthcare system. Chapter 4 examines the different types of work and when collaboration is important and when it is not. Chapter 5 describes three different types of interprofessional practice and how each weaves into the different types of work. Chapter 6 identifies some of the factors that shape when each type of interprofessional practice occurs and how practitioners engage in each type. Chapter 7 explains a common framework for how groups form and evolve. In healthcare, because groups are always changing, understanding where a group is in its evolution is critical for successful collaboration. Chapter 8 discusses how groups coordinate work through a concept called *group process*. This provides a framework for integrating the concepts introduced in preceding chapters with the evolving needs of patients.

The last six chapters of the book seek to build your skills in some specific areas that are important for better interprofessional practice. These chapters provide frameworks that you can transfer across healthcare settings and beyond. Chapter 9 defines different ways in which groups make decisions with a focus on the process of *consensus decision-making*. Chapter 10 examines hierarchy and power, including the different types of power and the importance of both leading and following. Chapter 11 discusses navigating conflict to find a solution that helps your patient and also does not undermining the group. Chapter 12 reviews how to give and receive feedback in order to improve your relationships with your colleagues and improve your overall collaboration. Chapter 13 discusses how to advocate for your perspective and work toward positive change. Finally, chapter 14 identifies how to build a community of collaborative practitioners to implement change focused on better health.

Each chapter starts with an introductory paragraph and objectives followed by some *initial reflection questions*. These questions are designed to get you thinking about the content area and ready to receive information about that area. Take these questions seriously, and you will get more out of this book.

The next section of each chapter presents the core material. We are in this section right now. The goal of this section is to provide content. For example, in this chapter, we have covered the rationale for interprofessional practice, introduced some terminology, and reviewed the structure of the book. My hope is to provide you with some new perspectives in manageable chunks that you can easily digest.

The following section of each chapter presents *application questions* related to the core material. These questions will usually have a right answer, though you may have to do some research to find that answer. The goal for this section is to work with the core material so you can see how it fits into the larger context of interprofessional practice. Throughout the book, I ask you to reflect upon your work as a healthcare practitioner. If you are currently a practitioner, you should answer these questions by thinking about your current work setting. But, if you are student, it's trickier. Try to answer these questions by envisioning your desired practice setting—you may need to pull on prior experiences to imagine what that setting might be like. The goal is for you to try to apply material to your experiences.

The next-to-last section of each chapter is *final reflection questions*. This is your chance to apply the material from the chapter to some of the challenges facing healthcare. I cannot give you the answers to these questions since the answers will depend on you and your context. The goal is for you to start to integrate the core material into your own individualized practice in the future. If you are using this book as part of a class, both these questions and the application questions are good for stimulating classroom discussion.

Finally, each chapter ends with some suggested reading and other resources. For example, in this chapter, I have covered very little of the history of interprofessional practice or interprofessional education, yet many people have been important advocates for this field over the past few decades. In addition, several documents have been published outlining competencies or approaches for interprofessional education. All of these publications have been important resources for the construction of this book, but I will not directly tie the sections of this book to any specific competency framework or educational approach. Instead, I provide a reference and description for each one in case you wish to examine them further.

A Confession

Please allow me a moment of frankness before I end this chapter. Over the past several years working in this field, I have learned much. Part of that learning process has involved making mistakes. As I have said, healthcare is complex and, as I have been unraveling this complexity, I have recognized that some of my long-held assumptions were wrong. The journey has been humbling, particularly as I have had to confront my biases. So, recognize me for who I am: a physician, an American, a practitioner and educator at a large academic center, a white male—all of these biases, and more, have shaped this book, sometimes in ways invisible to me. Throughout this book, I have endeavored to paint an accurate depiction of healthcare and collaboration. I am certain to have missed the mark at some points. In regard to these inevitable mistakes, I ask for two things: forgiveness and feedback. I won't promise to get everything right, but I will promise to try to make everything right in the future, with your help.

A Final Note on the Application of This Book

Health is about people. Health starts with the needs of people and their families and then engages many other individuals in the quest to improve or maintain health. People who shape the health of others are not just in healthcare; they are from fields such as education, social services, urban planning, law, government, and others. The strength of our society depends on how well these people collaborate. And the potential reached by our society in the future relies, in part, on how much better we will collaborate. Our imperative—and the impetus for this book—is to continue to build stronger collaborations that help people live better lives.

However, learning about collaboration is not just important for interprofessional work. Collaboration can also occur within a profession, which is known as *intraprofessional practice*. Conceptually, intraprofessional practice and interprofessional practice are similar. While we will touch on intraprofessional practice only a little, recognize that, in general, many of the principles are the same. Collaboration outside of work might actually be even more important. Friendships, romantic relationships, and family relations are all governed by the same concepts as interprofessional practice. While this book should certainly not be mistaken for a source of advice for the lovelorn, I will pull on non-healthcare examples to demonstrate points and encourage you to think about how these concepts might be applicable outside of the work environment. It's a big, complex world we live in, and hopefully this handbook will be a useful guide in many ways. I look forward to the adventure.

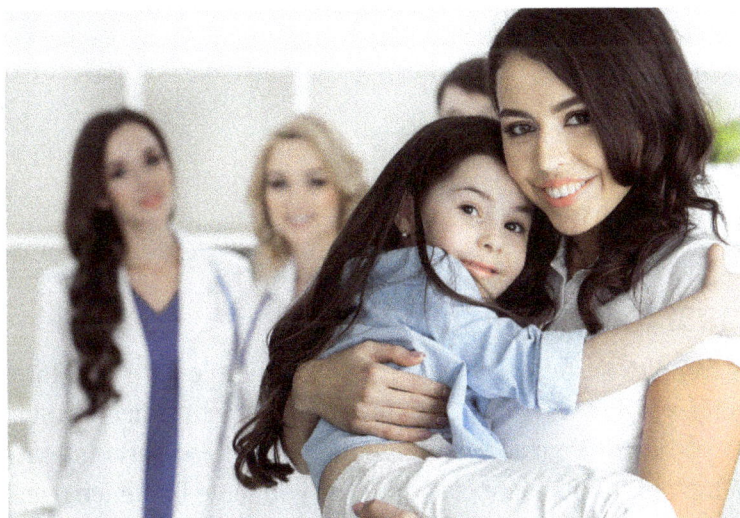

© Yellowj/Shutterstock.com

Application Questions

Based on your answers to the questions that started this chapter and the text above, what reasons would you give for improving interprofessional practice? Why is this an important area to study?

Describe two difficulties with using the term *healthcare system*.

Compare and contrast the use of the terms *healthcare practitioner*, *healthcare worker*, and *healthcare provider* in this book.

Describe two ways that the use of the term *patient* in this book might be imprecise or not completely accurate.

Final Reflection Questions

A complex system like healthcare has multiple parts that interact in varying ways. List as many parts of the healthcare system as you can. What factors determine how these parts interact? Which of these factors do you think you have influence over?

Based on your personal experience, can you think of occasions when you have seen poor health outcomes involving the following areas? What roles does better interprofessional practice have in addressing these challenges?

Poor Health Behaviors

Patient Safety

Health Equity

Wasteful or Inefficient Care

Care of Older Adults

In this book, I differentiate between healthcare workers and healthcare practitioners. What are some examples of essential contributions that healthcare workers who are not healthcare practitioners make to health outcomes? Healthcare workers who are not healthcare practitioners are less likely to receive specific training in interprofessional practice than healthcare practitioners. How should that influence how healthcare practitioners collaborate with these individuals?

We all have biases that stem from our life experience. What are some of the biases you might have based on your life experience? How might these biases affect your work in healthcare?

Further Reading

The *Framework for Action on Interprofessional Education and Collaborative Practice*, published by the World Health Organization (WHO), provides a global view of the need for better interprofessional practice and the role of training, especially interprofessional education, in creating a more collaborative workforce. Read this report online for free here: http://www.who.int/hrh/resources/framework_action/en/.

Discover other WHO resources related to interprofessional education at this link: http://whoeducationguidelines.org/blog/thematic-areas/interprofessional-education.

The National Academy of Medicine in the United States has published several important reports related to interprofessional education. You can access each report for free online. These include the following:

- The 2013 *Interprofessional Education for Collaboration: Learning How to Improve Health From Interprofessional Models Across the Continuum of Education to Practice—Workshop Summary*: http://nationalacademies.org/hmd/reports/2013/interprofessional-education-for-collaboration.aspx.
- The 2015 *Measuring the Impact of Interprofessional Education (IPE) on Collaborative Practice and Patient Outcomes* report: http://nationalacademies.org/hmd/reports/2015/impact-of-ipe.aspx.

Several groups have published recommended competencies for interprofessional education. While this book seeks to integrate all of them, each set of competencies differs. They are worth reviewing. Specifically:

- The U.S.-based Interprofessional Education Collaborative (IPEC) published its *Core Competencies for Interprofessional Collaborative Practice* in 2011 and updated those competencies in 2016. Find the IPEC competencies and other resources here: https://www.ipecollaborative.org/resources.html.
- The Canadian Interprofessional Health Collaborative (CIHC) published its *National Interprofessional Competency Framework* in 2010. This document and other resources are available here: https://www.cihc.ca/.

Several entities work across institutions to support interprofessional practice and education. The National Center for Interprofessional Practice and Education, https://nexusipe.org/, supports a predominantly U.S.-based community of individuals interested in these areas and curates a number of resources. Other regions of the world have similar organizations that you can access through the World Coordinating Committee sponsored by the World Health Organization, https://waipe.net/.

You can review a brief description of the determinants of health in the article "We Can Do Better—Improving the Health of the American People," which was authored by Steven Schroeder and published in the *New England Journal of Medicine* in 2007: http://www.nejm.org/doi/full/10.1056/NEJMsa073350. Schroeder also wrote about the continued dangers of cigarette smoking in "New Evidence That Cigarette Smoking Remains the Most Important Health Hazard," a 2013 article in the *New England Journal of Medicine*: http://www.nejm.org/doi/full/10.1056/NEJMe1213751.

Learn about the aging population from a global perspective in "An Aging World: 2015" published by the U.S. Census Bureau in 2016: https://www.census.gov/content/dam/Census/library/publications/2016/demo/p95-16-1.pdf.

Finally, the Center on Society and Health at my institution, Virginia Commonwealth University, has done some great work funded by the Robert Wood Johnson Foundation that describes the differences in life expectancy in a number of U.S. cities. View that project and the maps of these cities here: https://societyhealth.vcu.edu/work/the-projects/mapping-life-expectancy.html.

SECTION 2

The Individual Practitioner

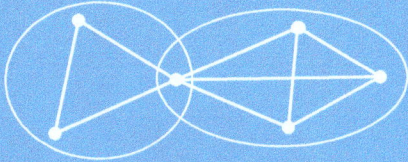

CHAPTER 2

Professions and Scopes of Practice

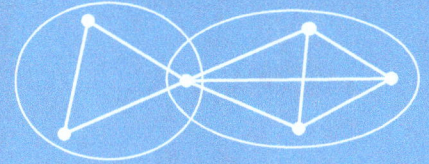

In this chapter and the next, we will talk about the concepts of professions, scopes of practice, professional roles, and individual responsibilities. These concepts define who we are in the healthcare system, our professional activities—what we do—and how we fit together. This chapter will begin to explore these concepts by defining a profession and the concept of scope of practice. By the end of this chapter, you will be able to:

▸ describe what defines a profession,
▸ explain the concept of scope of practice and its relationship to licensure, and
▸ identify how the concepts of professions and scopes of practice influence collaboration and interprofessional practice.

Initial Reflection Questions

You likely have an intuitive sense of what a profession is, but how does a profession actually define itself? What differentiates someone who has a profession from someone who has a job?

How does having participants from different professions support collaboration? How can professional differences make collaboration challenging?

The Spheres of Professional Activities

People from different health professions are the fundamental units of interprofessional practice; think of them as the raw ingredients in the magic stew that we are trying to make. We need to know what these ingredients are before we can start combining them together.

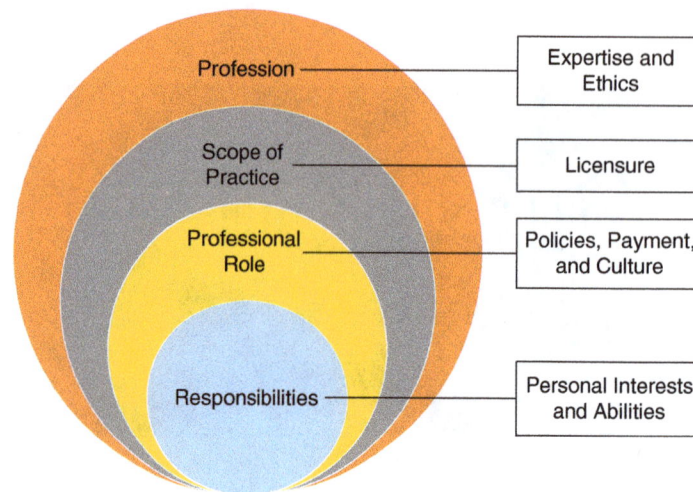

Figure 2.1 The Spheres of Professional Activities. Source: Alan Dow.

The basic units of work for these different healthcare practitioners are *professional activities*. Healthcare practitioners perform many different types of professional activities, ranging from counseling and interviewing patients to performing invasive surgical procedures and administering potentially toxic therapies. Many factors shape which professional activities a specific individual performs.

To help you think about the professional activities of each profession, we will use a framework for the different spheres that define professional activities (see Figure 2.1). These spheres are nested within each other, with the outermost sphere being how a profession defines itself, the next sphere being scope of practice, the next sphere being professional role, and the smallest sphere being responsibilities. An individual's professional activities typically reside in this smallest sphere of responsibilities, but professional activities are not limited to a job's current responsibilities. Over the next two chapters, we will explore each of these spheres, the factors that determine them, and their effects on interprofessional practice.

Understanding Professions as a Foundation

If you are reading this text, you are almost certainly part of a profession. But what does that mean? How do professions come about, and what separates a profession from other types of work? Let's look at the defining characteristics of a profession.

- **Expertise:** Members of a profession share a specific area of expertise. They have some knowledge or skills that the rest of society lacks.
- **Education and training:** To develop this expertise, individuals who aspire to join a profession require education and training.
- **Ethics:** Because of their expertise, members of a profession often have power over individuals accessing professional services. Professionals must therefore adhere to some sort of code of ethics to prevent the possibility of taking advantage of these individuals.
- **Licensure:** Finally, to assure society that the aspiring professional is ready to work independently after training and comply with the ethical duties of the profession, professions require some sort of licensure. Note that the concept of licensure is tricky because it also defines a profession's scope of practice. We'll differentiate between a profession and a scope of practice in a moment.

Every profession is built on the bedrock of these four characteristics. A profession is a group of people who have specialized expertise, developed through education and training, governed by an ethical code, and endorsed by licensure. Some sort of professional organization, such as an accreditor or licensing board, oversees the training and licensure process to ensure that members of the profession meet standards of expertise and ethics.

Professions are diverse. In my state, you can be licensed in over 50 different professions, ranging from athletic trainers to nursing home administrators. Cosmetologists, equine dental technicians, embalmers, and massage therapists need licenses too. Think about all of those different kinds of expertise. While not all of these professionals provide health services, it's tough to draw a line around which professions constitute the health professions. Realizing that the professions are diverse, you can be open to all sorts of potential collaborations (see sidebar).

A Pharmacist Walks Into a Barbershop

One well-documented health disparity in the United States is the rate of blood-pressure control. Black men have worse rates of blood-pressure control than white men or women of either race. One related factor seems to be that black men see healthcare practitioners less frequently than the other groups. However, many people who don't visit their primary care practitioners frequently still get regular haircuts.

So, a group of barbers and pharmacists partnered to take on this health challenge. The barbers encouraged their clients to meet with a pharmacist at the barbershop for a blood-pressure assessment and possible medication therapy. After six months, the clients who started the study with uncontrolled hypertension and had been treated by the pharmacists were five times more likely to have controlled their blood pressure. That's how you feel as good as you look.

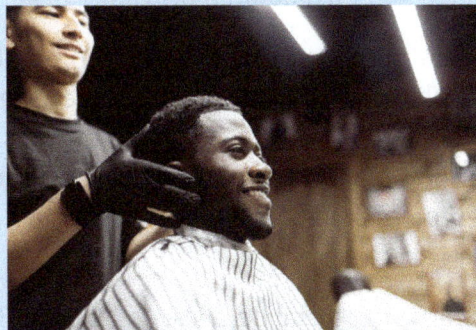

© Pressmaster/Shutterstock.com

This definition of a profession is not perfect. Many areas of deep expertise require lots of training yet don't require a license. For example, most professors and researchers would be considered professionals, yet they are unlicensed. Business leaders, including hospital CEOs, may be responsible for thousands of employees and billions of dollars of economic activity, yet they don't need a license. And there's no license for being a politician or high-ranking governmental official. Granted, sometimes there are credentials that support someone's expertise in a given arena (like having obtained a Ph.D. in a scientific field), but some people who would seem to be professionals fall outside this definition.

Also, consider how tradesmen like auto mechanics compare to our definition of a profession. Rarely do I feel as helpless as when I take my car to be serviced and a mechanic tells me that I need a repair that will cost several hundred dollars. (I can imagine this is how my patients must sometimes feel.) I have no clue whether the mechanic is being honest, but I usually submit to the mechanic's recommendation. I presume the mechanic is being ethical. But are auto mechanics part of a profession? Technically, no, though many of the principles underlying our definition apply.

The definition of a profession begins to help us think about the people we collaborate with, but it is imperfect. The clerical and custodial staff in healthcare aren't part of a profession, yet they are essential to providing health services. Think of understanding different professions as a starting point for beginning to understand collaboration in healthcare, but recognize that it is not the whole story.

Evolution of Professions in Health

One reason that defining professions can be challenging is because they evolve. Let's put some historical context around professions. That helps to explain how we define professions today and how that definition has evolved to create some of the tension around professions today. Not to dwell too much on physicians, but this profession is the classic example, so let's briefly look at the evolution of the physician profession.

Around 1900, physicians, osteopaths, apothecaries (future pharmacists), and others all diagnosed and treated ailments. The quality of care was lousy. There were literal snake oil salesmen, many of whom described themselves as part of any or all of these "health" professions. To improve the quality of care, physicians, with the support of the public and governmental officials, established the doctor of medicine license with defined training and ethics. Over a few years, this profession, with government support, pushed out the other practitioners who had previously diagnosed and treated ailments. In the process, physicians ascended to the top of the medical hierarchy in terms of both prestige and income from providing health services.

But this ascension was not without a cost to society as a whole. Accessing health services became more challenging as medical care became less available and more expensive. And physicians were often not good partners in trying to solve these challenges. While the physician profession evolved because there was a societal need to ensure expertise, the physician profession took advantage of this professionalization to exert authority, exclude other practitioners, and create barriers for people seeking services.

Fast-forward several decades, and we faced a shortage of practitioners who could diagnose and treat ailments in primary care. We needed practitioners in addition to physicians to fill this need. Fortunately, the evolution of the physician profession provided a template for the professionalization of other fields. Over the past few decades, an increasing number of professions with advanced training and licensure have emerged to diagnose and treat ailments. Most people, including most physicians, agree that this is a good thing for society overall.

This is emblematic of the challenge facing us: we need to ensure that society has the expertise it needs and, to do that, we need cooperation across professions to deliver health services in the best way. This is where interprofessional practice fits. Interprofessional practice seeks to leverage expertise while sharing authority and responsibility for health across professions.

Scope of Practice

While defining a profession can be challenging, the definition of scope of practice is clearer. Scope of practice is the concept of what a practitioner is allowed to do under the terms of

Nurse Anesthesia: A Case Study in Successful Professional Evolution

While nurses have been involved in anesthesia since the practice began in the mid-1800s, nurse anesthesia certification has only existed for about 60 years. It took almost a hundred years to recognize that the capacity for nurses to anesthetize and wake an operative patient successfully required extra training.

Now, a nurse anesthetist must complete a bachelor of science degree in nursing and an additional two to three years of training to become a certified registered nurse anesthetist. This licensure ensures surgical patients that, while they are in the most vulnerable of all positions, they are being cared for by well-qualified healthcare practitioners. Nurse anesthetists are involved in almost all surgeries and have superlative outcomes. Nurse anesthetists also work all over the world, including in some of the areas most lacking in health services. Nurse anesthesia is a profession that was created over the past century and has grown into being essential in healthcare.

his or her license. Can that individual administer medication? Write a prescription? Perform an invasive procedure? Scope of practice answers these questions.

Scope of practice is a legal concept, meaning it is either defined by laws or defined by legally designated entities, like state boards. Scope of practice defines the professional activities that a licensed healthcare professional can legally perform in a certain geographic area such as a state or country. While licensure is part of the definition of a profession, your education and expertise may prepare you to do more than you are licensed to do in a particular geographic area. Your licensure sets the legal limit for your scope of practice.

The scope of practice defined by a license would seem to be pretty standard, but that is not the case. Licensure varies. In the United States, the criteria for licensure can differ by state. Nurse practitioners, for example, can practice independently in most states, but some states require nurse practitioners to have a collaborating physician. (Greater independence of nurse practitioners from physicians is the national trend, supported by studies of outcomes.) Another common example is heterogeneous continuing education requirements by states. While my state requires 60 continuing education credits every two years to renew my medical license, the number and timing of these credits differ greatly by state. While states often defer to a national entity for testing such as board exams, they set their own standards in other areas.

> **Nonsensical Variations in Training**
>
> Between different professions, there are variations in scope of practice that don't make much sense. An example is training for medication-assisted treatment (MAT). As you know, we are in the midst of a crisis of opiate use disorders. One of the best treatments for opiate use disorders is MAT, which combines the prescribed medication buprenorphine (Suboxone) with counseling and social support. Prescribing buprenorphine is not especially risky, but, according to federal law in the United States, practitioners need special training to learn how to follow protocols for buprenorphine prescribing.
>
> Here's the nonsensical part: according to these federal regulations, physicians need eight hours of training to prescribe buprenorphine, while nurse practitioners or physician's assistants need 24 hours of training! This variation in training requirements between professions makes no sense. I can assure you that the average physician is worse at following protocols than a NP, PA, or pharmacist. And physicians are generally not better trained to treat addiction. This nonsensical variation in training adds an additional barrier to providing needed care to individuals with substance use disorders.

Scope of practice can vary within a geographic area for other reasons. While practitioners in my city are generally governed by Virginia law, practitioners working at the Veterans Affairs (VA) medical center are governed by federal law. The differences between Virginia and federal scopes of practice are small, but they can be important. Pharmacists who prescribe medications at a VA hospital are listed as the prescriber, while elsewhere in my city, under the state scope of practice, a collaborating physician must be listed as the prescriber. Lab ordering functions similarly. As a result, it is much easier for pharmacists to track their patients and ensure high-quality care within the VA.

Scope of practice begins to define the professional activities of a healthcare professional. Just keep in mind that the scope of practice and profession are not synonymous and that scope does not define the specific professional activities of an individual.

Specialization

One specific element of professions worth highlighting is *specialization*. Specialization is the concept of a profession being internally divided into subprofessions or specialties. Most professions have

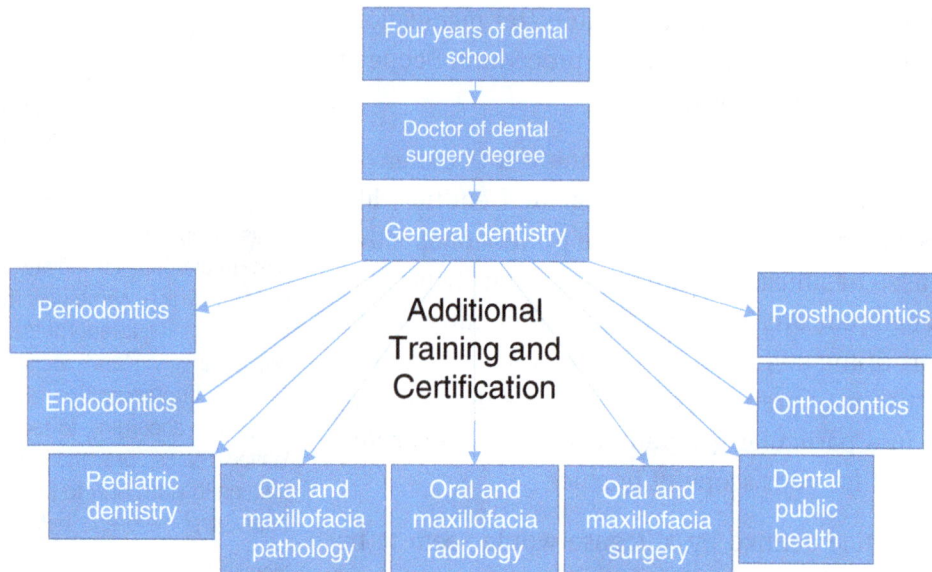

Figure 2.2 Pathways to Specialization for Dentistry in the United States. Most dentists are general dentists, but practitioners in this field can undergo additional training to receive certification as a specialist in any of nine different areas. Source: Alan Dow.

some degree of specialization. For example, the American Dental Association recognizes nine dental specialties (see Figure 2.2).

Specialties start as informal differentiations in interest and expertise. As these differentiations become more formalized with specific training and licensure, they become what could be considered a new profession with a new scope of practice.

Specialization can lead to intraprofessional conflict. For instance, palliative care is an interprofessional field with practitioners from many fields. Within the specialization structure of physicians, palliative care might be housed within a department of oncology, geriatrics, primary care, or some other traditional specialty. While this intraprofessional heterogeneity of physicians involved in palliative care can provide important diversity, it may also lead to conflict within an institution or across the field. This has led some institutions to create centers or departments of palliative care to leverage this diversity and resolve these conflicts. Recognize that specialization can cause intraprofessional problems similar to those we see interprofessionally.

Scope of Practice and Interprofessional Collaboration

Let's wrap up this chapter by looking at how scopes of practice interact during interprofessional collaboration and how you should integrate this concept into your professional work.

First, it's important to understand the scope of practice of your own profession. You may be getting a limited view in your current setting. If you are new to your profession, spend time speaking with mentors and interacting with colleagues through professional organizations to understand the breadth of your profession and the extent of your scope of practice. Be on the lookout for changes, like new laws, that may affect your profession's scope of practice. Professions grow and change, so don't let the past limit your own professional identity.

Second, you will work with some professions more often than others. As you work with individuals from these professions, work to understand their scopes of practice. I recommend approaching this question from two directions:

1. **Ask individuals about their profession.** People are usually happy to talk about their work. They may have insights about how they wish their field would change, and you may be able to help them work differently. In addition, most people love to talk about themselves, and being curious about their work will build your relationship with them.

2. **Read about how professional organizations define their scopes of their practice.** Sometimes, individuals aren't aware of the full extent of their own scope of practice. Professions evolve, and your colleagues may not be aware of how their profession is changing. Be curious, especially as you start to think about how to collaborate better.

Third, think about how your profession's scope of practice fits together with the scopes of practice of your colleagues from other professions. Undoubtedly, there will be areas where professional activities intersect. For example, who should educate a patient about a health condition? In the next chapter, we will talk about why one profession might be better positioned than another to educate a patient, even if both professions have patient education in their scopes of practice.

Of course, these activities that cross scopes of practice don't have to be an either/or situation. The best care is delivered when we work together—in our example, when each profession is involved in patient education that is relevant to its work and reinforces the messages from other practitioners. While a physician might make a diagnosis and outline the therapeutic options and prognosis for a patient, a nurse might expand on that information by working with patient-defined concerns to individualize education and provide more patient-centered care. A pharmacist might then focus on medications and their side effects and optimal timing for ingestion with food or other medications, while therapists work to integrate a treatment plan into the practicalities of a patient's daily life. The goal is to be complementary to each other to strengthen care overall.

Scopes of practice can also have a dark side: they can be the source of professional conflict. Imagine if the physician in this example made a minor error—let's say by prescribing a twice-a-day medication when a once-a-day medication was available. Would other practitioners speak up, or would they doubt themselves and not feel like those decisions were part of their own scopes of practice? Or what if, because of overlap in scopes of practice, everyone assumed the patient was being educated by someone else so that the patient never learned about the medication? You can imagine how scope of practice might hamper patient care. Better interprofessional collaboration is the answer to these types of issues.

Application Questions

Consider your own profession. How would you describe what your profession does? What is or will be your scope of practice? Use the links at the end of this chapter and the board of licensure in your locality (your state, in the United States) to supplement your answer.

Think about three professions that closely collaborate with your profession. How would you describe the scopes of practice of these professions? Use the links at the end of this chapter and other web resources to supplement your answer. What do you see as areas of overlap in your future work?

Profession 1:
  Scope

  Areas of overlap

Profession 2:
  Scope

  Areas of overlap

Profession 3:
  Scope

  Areas of overlap

Reflection Questions

Based on the areas of overlap between your profession and the other professions that you listed above, how will you work to ensure that you and your colleagues from other professions complement each other? What are some approaches to ensure collaborative care and limit conflict?

Identify a recent or pending change in your profession's scope of practice. (Searching your professional organization's website may help.) Why did this change occur? How might this change help patients? How might it create overlap with other professions?

Can you identify any areas of variation in your profession's scope of practice across different geographic areas? How might this variation influence patient outcomes? Practitioners' satisfaction with their practices? The desirability of practicing in a certain geographic area?

Further Reading

The System of Professions: An Essay on the Division of Expert Labor by Andrew Abbott is an excellent place to start if you want to read more about the theories of why professions exist, how professions have evolved, and what forces have driven professionalization.

The Social Transformation of American Medicine by Paul Starr describes the evolution of medicine in the United States. While Starr's primary focus is physicians, the book covers the development of professions in general, the business of medicine, and the impact of these changes on society as a whole.

Listed below are the professional organizations that compose the Interprofessional Education Collaborative (IPEC) in the United States. These organizations' websites provide one perspective on how each profession defines itself; they may be useful for completing the work in this chapter or for reference in the future.

The Academy of Nutrition and Dietetics (ACEND) is available at https://www.eatrightpro.org/acend.

The American Association of Colleges of Nursing (AACN) is available at http://www.aacnnursing.org.

The National League for Nursing (NLN) is available at http://www.nln.org.

Note that nursing has two academic professional organizations, both of which are involved in accreditation, advocacy, and continuing professional development.

The American Association of Colleges of Osteopathic Medicine (AACOM) is available at https://www.aacom.org.

The Association of American Medical Colleges (AAMC) is available at https://www.aamc.org.

Graduates from both osteopathic schools (AACOM) and allopathic medical schools (AAMC) function as physicians in the healthcare system.

The American Association of Colleges of Pharmacy (AACP) is available at https://www.aacp.org.

The American Association of Colleges of Podiatric Medicine (AACPM) is available at http://www.aacpm.org.

The American Occupational Therapy Association (AOTA) is available at https://www.aota.org.

The American Council of Academic Physical Therapy (ACAPT) is available at http://www.acapt.org.

The American Dental Education Association (ADEA) is available at http://www.adea.org.

The American Psychological Association (APA) is available at http://www.apa.org.

The American Speech-Language-Hearing Association (ASHA) is available at https://www.asha.org.

The Association of Academic Health Sciences Libraries (AAHSL) is available at https://www.aahsl.org.

The Association of American Veterinary Medical Colleges (AAVMC) is available at http://www.aavmc.org.

There is debate about whether interprofessional practice should focus primarily on human health. I have included veterinarians for completeness and because their practice is relevant to human health when it comes to zoonoses (diseases transmitted between humans and animals), policy in areas like appropriate antibiotic use, and the benefits of human-animal interaction on mental health.

The Association of Chiropractic Colleges (ACC) is available at http://www.chirocolleges.org.

The Association of Schools and Colleges of Optometry (ASCO) is available at https://optometriceducation.org.

The Association of Schools and Programs of Public Health (ASPPH) is available at https://www.aspph.org.

The Association of Schools of Allied Health Professions (ASAHP) is available at http://www.asahp.org.

The Council on Social Work Education (CSWE) is available at https://www.cswe.org.

The Physician Assistant Education Association (PAEA) is available at http://paeaonline.org.

To read more about pharmacists collaborating with barbers, see Ronald Victor and colleagues' article "A Cluster-Randomized Trial of Blood-Pressure Reduction in Black Barbershops" in *The New England Journal of Medicine* from 2018.

CHAPTER 3

Roles and Responsibilities

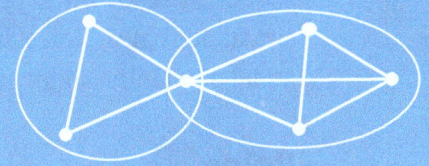

What we do—our professional activities—is usually a fraction of our profession's capabilities. While a profession's definition of itself and its scope of practice as authorized by a license specify what a professional could do, neither describes what a specific person within a profession usually does. Instead, we work in professional settings within a professional role with more limited professional responsibilities. This limitation in our scope of practice is not a bad thing: it helps us focus, develop expertise, and, hopefully, engage in professional activities that we find personally meaningful. That is not to say that our responsibilities are static—they change based on many factors. By the end of this chapter, you will be able to:

▸ define professional roles and professional responsibilities,
▸ identify some of the drivers of professional roles and responsibilities, and
▸ describe how responsibilities can be complementary between or shared by multiple practitioners.

Initial Reflection Questions

Think about your ideal job. What are some of the professional activities that you would like to perform during a typical workday?

What about professional activities that are in your professional scope of practice but that you would rather not perform during a typical day?

What factors determine the professional activities within your scope of practice that you would or would not perform during a typical day? How might those factors shape your choice of a job?

Roles and Responsibilities

As we have seen, the scope of practice, as defined by licensure, outlines the legal limits of a professional's activities. However, just because an individual professional can legally do anything within a certain scope of practice does not mean that person actually performs all of the activities within that scope. Instead, most professionals' job responsibilities represent a subset of their possible professional activities. Roles and responsibilities are often lumped together, but they are not the same thing, so let's examine them separately.

Roles

Think of your *professional role* as your title within a setting: you may be "the occupational therapist," "the audiologist," or "the physician's assistant." Roles are labels that imply a scope of practice and expertise in a certain set of professional activities. But the professional activities in a specific role are usually not as broad as an entire scope of practice because professional role is shaped in part by scope of practice and in part by culture.

To contrast professional role and scope of practice, let's look at an example. While most healthcare practitioners receive some training in their foundational education in both pediatrics and geriatrics, most healthcare practitioners care for either children or older adults, but not both. If you work at an elementary school or a children's hospital, you will rarely use your training in geriatrics; likewise, most nursing homes do not have pediatric patients.

For some professions, these professional roles require special training and certification in pediatrics or geriatrics. This formalized expertise is similar to scope of practice. For other professions, these professional roles are not formalized, and individuals develop practical expertise as they work with a specific population. The overarching point is that a professional role defines some area of expertise within a scope of practice; the population that you work with is just one factor that defines your role and expertise.

While scope of practice shrinks into a role based on the population served, culture adds variation across similar populations. *Culture* is the way things are done in a particular place. That place may be big or small: a country, locality, institution, clinical unit, or specific group of practitioners. Culture may be shaped by formal rules or policies (for example, scope of practice) or may be defined by subtler, unwritten manifestations of relationships. Culture and cultural norms are themes throughout this book; for now, let's just think of culture as the way things are done in a particular place and recognize that professional roles are a blend of culture and scope of practice.

An example of the impact of culture on professional roles is variability in how care is delivered between units; sometimes, neighboring units within a single institution have very different ways of providing care. Why this variation exists is often unclear, particularly when one approach is clearly superior. Something in the culture is shaping the work of these practitioners. Variation can be good or bad—having typical ways of doing things is usually a positive, as it keeps everyone on the same page, but variation can also lead to innovation and positive change. Keep your eyes open for variation and think about how culture is shaping professional roles and influencing collaboration.

Beyond scope of practice and culture, professional roles can be shaped by many other factors, such as new research and changes in reimbursement. The sidebar describes shifting pharmacist roles; other professions are undergoing similar changes. For example, physical therapists are working in primary

The Slow Adoption of Pharmacist-Led Chronic Disease Management

A number of studies have shown that pharmacists are superior to typical primary care physicians in managing chronic health conditions like diabetes and hypertension and in monitoring long-term anti-coagulation with warfarin. Pharmacists excel at understanding medication options, counseling patients about how to take medication and what side effects to expect, and navigating the formularies of pharmacies and insurers. This makes sense considering the scope of practice of pharmacists. In addition, pharmacists tend to be more accessible and see patients more frequently. Compared to a community-based pharmacist, a typical primary care practitioner is more difficult to see face-to-face and has many other patient care tasks to address other than chronic disease management. Not surprisingly, pharmacists achieve clinical goals for chronic disease management at higher rates than typical primary care doctors.

Yet, pharmacists have been slow to take up the role of chronic disease management. Why?

To start, pharmacists need the right training to be effective in this role. Not every pharmacist has the expertise to evaluate and manage patients with chronic disease. Pharmacy schools and residencies are working to build this expertise, but that takes time. So, limitations in the workforce are one issue.

Another issue is that, in some states, licensure does not grant pharmacists the independence necessary for pharmacist-led chronic disease management to work. Some critical professional activities may not be in their scope of practice, at least in a fashion that is easily implemented (i.e., not requiring excessive physician supervision). An overly restrictive scope of practice can get in the way regardless of what the evidence says.

In addition, some insurers don't pay for pharmacists to perform chronic disease management activities. In a perverse but common twisting of incentives, it is costlier to invest in chronic disease management up front. Because the consequences of unmanaged chronic disease, like heart attacks and strokes, might happen years later, the insurance company's bottom line favors less early care, especially if the patient could change insurance before these costlier medical problems occur. Reimbursement drives adoption of this role.

Lastly, primary care practitioners (PCPs) have been slow to adapt to this approach. Many PCPs did not have interprofessional education in school and were not trained to collaborate with pharmacists in this way. Some may also worry that pharmacists will assume full responsibility for chronic disease management, which accounts for a large segment of primary care visits. While we all want the best for our patients, our individual abilities and interests shape collaboration, and that's not always for the best.

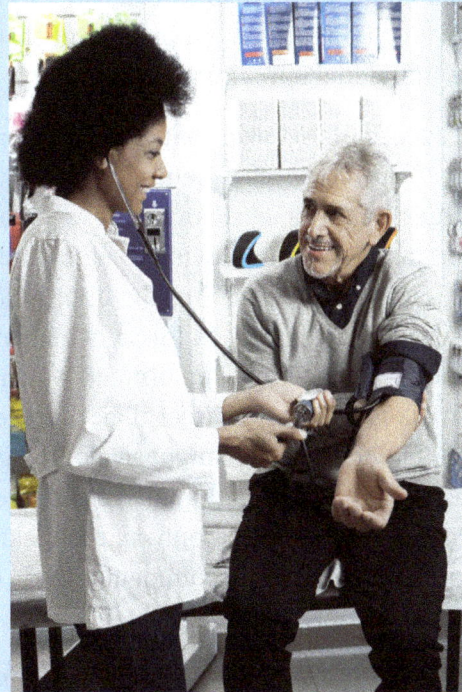

care practices to prevent falls, and occupational therapists are trying to help patients better manage their medications. Professional roles evolve, yet even when these new roles are evidence-based and effective, they need to be rewarded financially and supported by other professions to be integrated into the culture of how we deliver care.

Responsibilities

Responsibilities are the professional activities that an individual does as part of a professional role. These are granular units of work like taking a blood pressure, documenting notes in an electronic health record, or talking to a patient's family members. In total, responsibilities define a role. Some activities are specific to certain professions, while others may be shared by multiple professions. Like roles, responsibilities change based on a variety of factors, and who is responsible for a professional activity may also shift. Because of these changes, having a shared understanding of who is responsible for each professional activity and which roles can perform an activity is essential for providing the best care, especially as the needs of patients and the constraints on your colleagues evolve.

To examine the connection between scope of practice, roles, and responsibilities, let's look at speech-language pathology. Licensure as a speech-language pathologist defines the maximum scope of practice for these practitioners. But that scope of practice is much broader than the typical practice of an individual speech-language pathologist.

One speech-language pathologist might work in an acute care setting, performing activities such as evaluating the swallowing function of an individual who had a recent stroke or identifying the appropriate diet and feeding approach for someone with functional or cognitive impairment. Much of this work is diagnostic rather than therapeutic. Often, the speech-language pathologist in this setting works with patients for a very short duration, perhaps only once, making an assessment and recommendations for others to carry forward.

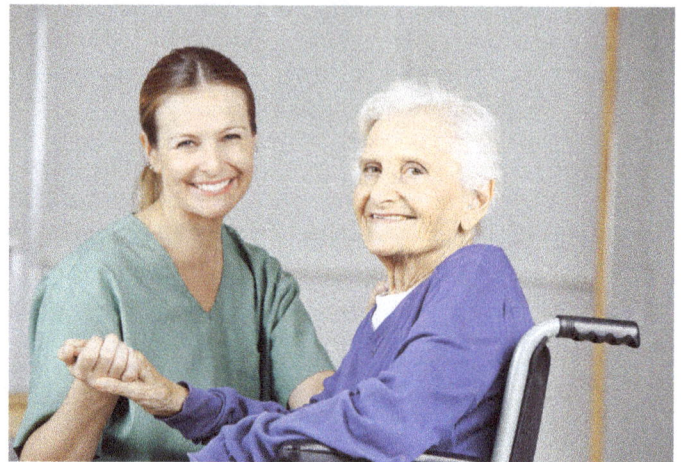

© Robert Kneschke/Shutterstock.com

Another speech-language pathologist might work in a rehabilitation setting where professional activities include working with patients to improve vocalization, feeding, and other activities. Here, the work is more therapeutic and less diagnostic. The rehabilitative speech-language pathologist works with patients over a longer term, usually weeks or months, and has the opportunity to build relationships with patients as they work to regain and maximize function over time.

Still another speech-language pathologist might work with children in schools, enhancing clarity and quality of speech production or assessing children with learning difficulties. There are more opportunities for diagnosis here than in a rehabilitation setting, and this individual may have the most longitudinal relationship with his or her patients (or clients) as they strive to achieve the most normal function possible.

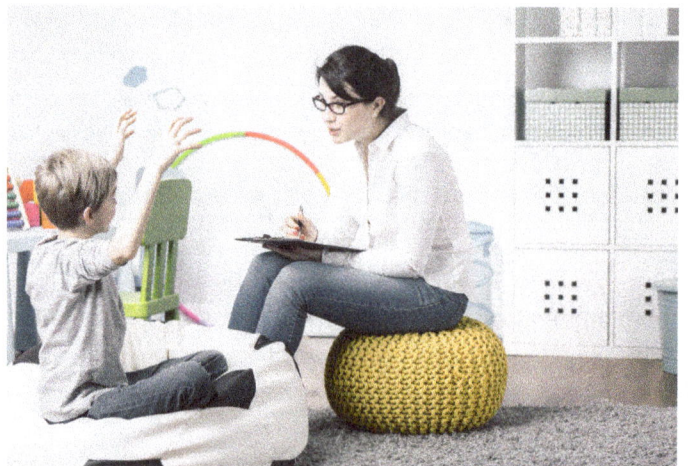

© Photographee.eu/Shutterstock.com

You can see how, within the profession of speech-language pathology, the setting and the patient population lead to dramatically different roles and professional responsibilities. A similar spectrum of roles and responsibilities can be seen in many healthcare professions. A critical care nurse engages in different activities from a nurse in a clinic, one performing home visits, or one in a school. A primary care doctor has different professional activities from a surgeon or radiologist. And a pharmacist may work in a hospital, drugstore, governmental agency, or pharmaceutical company, each of which brings with it different roles and responsibilities. While the profession and scope of practice are useful labels, they do not begin to describe the responsibilities of a specific role.

Turning Professional Activities into Professional Responsibilities

In the last chapter, I stated that individuals' professional activities are the fundamental units of healthcare and that our job was to mix these activities together to best meet the needs of patients. So, how do we turn these professional activities into responsibilities that will allow us to provide the best care? For the rest of the book, we will focus on what collaboration is, what shapes collaboration, and how to collaborate better. But, before we leave individuals, let's look at some of the drivers of individual responsibilities.

Driver 1: The Needs of Patients

At the center of healthcare is, of course, the patient. Imagine that you are performing your typical day-to-day roles and responsibilities on an uneventful day. Suddenly, a patient becomes acutely ill. You and your colleagues must adapt to help that patient. You might assess the patient. Or you might provide some stabilizing treatment. Or maybe you go find more help.

That's a dramatic example, but the point is that responsibilities are dynamic. Patients have different needs, and responsibilities must shift to best meet the changing needs of each patient. One patient may need a more thorough assessment, while another may need extensive counseling and education. Some patients are straightforward; others are not. Within your entire scope of practice, the primary driver of your responsibilities is your patients.

Driver 2: Setting

Setting also shapes roles and responsibilities. Compare working in a high-tech, academic medical center with working in a hospital in a rural community or even a developing country. Factors like the availability of professional expertise, technology, and therapeutics shape responsibilities. In a large academic medical center, there is often someone with specialized expertise to ask for help, but, in other settings, you may be the lone expert. In settings with lesser resources, you can make a tremendous impact, but you may also feel in over your head. Your responsibilities may be closer to your full scope of practice.

Time of day is also a factor. Even in our most advanced hospitals, fewer resources and personnel are available at night or on weekends. If you are working during an "off" time, you will likely find yourself with greater responsibilities and less backup.

As we saw above, different settings have different cultures. While technology, staffing, and time of day shape both responsibilities and culture, culture is a complex manifestation of all aspects of a setting and can be described by each individual's professional responsibilities. Culture defines responsibilities.

Driver 3: Regulations

Another factor that can determine roles and responsibilities is the applicability of regulations such as policies, rules, or laws. The activities of healthcare professionals are often shaped by rules outside the immediate setting. Some of these regulations may be directly linked to licensure and scope of practice. For example, only certain professions can pronounce an individual deceased or fill out a death certificate. Rules around reimbursement are regulations, including who can get reimbursed for a professional activity, which medication are on a formulary, and what procedures are paid for by insurance. Many other responsibilities are defined by rules or policies within a specific setting of care (see sidebar).

Who Collects the Best Medication History?

Medication reconciliation is one of the most important tasks in the care of complex patients. *Medication reconciliation* means identifying the correct list of medications that a patient is taking, including dose, route, and frequency. This task can be challenging because many patients have trouble remembering all the details of their medications, and the list in a medical office or fill record in a pharmacy may be inaccurate, especially if patients see multiple prescribers and use multiple pharmacies.

As patients move between different settings such as the clinic, the hospital, and home, an incorrect medication list is a big source of errors. Important medications can be omitted; new medications can interact with old, unreported medications; and medication classes can be duplicated. Regulators, like the Joint Commission that oversees hospital accreditation, have rules requiring effective medication reconciliation.

At my hospital, we particularly struggled with medication reconciliation when a patient was admitted to the hospital from the emergency department. Initially, our policy designated the admitting physicians as solely responsible. Since physicians took a medication history from the patient on admission, this made sense.

However, over several years, we had several significant errors due to inaccurate medication reconciliation. It turned out that physicians were too busy addressing the patient's overall presenting medical condition to carefully review the medication list. In addition, they did not have access to all the records, such as information from pharmacies and primary care offices.

In response, leaders at my hospital pulled together an interprofessional group to figure out a better approach. This group devised a new policy for medication reconciliation that, with the support of leadership, included hiring several pharmacy technicians solely focused on medication reconciliation. Pharmacy technicians are experts in medications, including what they look like. When a patient says he or she takes "a pink pill," pharmacy technicians are much better than most other practitioners at identifying this medication.

The pharmacy technicians worked in the emergency department with the patients admitted to the hospital. They had the responsibility of ascertaining the most accurate medication list possible from the patient and the patient's pharmacy and other practitioners. Then, they entered this list in the patient's electronic health record as historical medications that the medical team could then easily convert to the right inpatient and outpatient medication orders. Carving out these responsibilities in a new role helped the admitting medical team function more efficiently, reduced errors, and improved patient care.

Driver 4: Collaborators

The final driver is our colleagues. The whole point of this book is that we do not practice in isolation, so, of course, our colleagues shape our responsibilities. Professional activities can affect how we interact with colleagues in a couple of ways (see Figure 3.1).

Some activities are complementary but not shared. In this case, neither person performs the other's professional activity, but they depend on each other. An example is a scrub nurse and a surgeon in an operating room. The nurse is solely responsible for some activities, like ensuring proper conditions of instrumentation, and the surgeon is solely responsible for other activities, like making an incision. If something is wrong with the instrumentation or the incision, both individuals may need to adapt their activities. They are closely interdependent, but each professional has his or her own professional responsibilities.

Contrast complementary activities with shared activities. Here, there is overlap in the ability to complete an activity. Monitoring blood pressure is an example. Many professions have that activity in their scope of practice, but which individual is responsible may depend on many factors including some of those listed above. A medical assistant might typically take a blood pressure reading in a primary care office, but if the medical assistant is busy with other tasks or if the reading is clinically complex (perhaps for an obese patient or an orthostatic patient), a primary care practitioner may complete that activity. Communication between colleagues is essential for defining who is responsible and how responsibilities fit together to best deliver care.

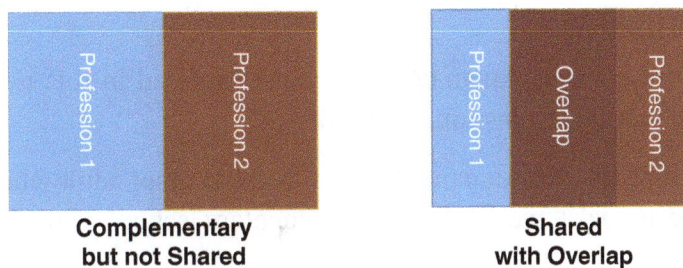

Figure 3.1 Professional Responsibilities as Complementary or Overlapping. Source: Alan Dow.

Roles, Responsibilities, and Your Career

If you are a student, an important consideration for your future career is the responsibilities of a specific role. While licensure will allow you a broad scope of practice, you will need to consider which responsibilities and activities you wish to perform under that scope of practice. Are there professional activities you really enjoy? Are there others you would prefer to avoid?

In addition, some activities require further training that falls short of licensure. Certifications in wound care, diabetes education, or hand therapy are examples. As you think about your ideal job, recognize the range of professional activities in your profession. Use that knowledge as you consider job prospects and future training so that, someday, you can have a professional role that you will love.

Application Questions

Think about your own ideal role. What are some of that role's professional activities that will be influenced by each of the following drivers? Try to think about activities you might or might not do based on aspects of each of the categories below.

Patient needs

Setting

Regulations

Collaborators

For the activities you listed above, which are shared responsibilities with other professions, and which are complementary responsibilities that are not shared?

Questions for Discussion

Consider the example of the speech-language pathologist explored in this chapter. Using the chart below, compare and contrast the professional activities of:

- a speech-language pathologist working in a hospital with an older adult who just had a stroke and
- a speech-language pathologist working in an elementary school with a child with a speech impediment.

Describe the similarities and differences in their work. Think about the types of professional activities they might do in terms of patient needs, setting (including available resources and impact of culture), regulations, and collaborators.

	Hospital-based speech-language pathologist	School-based speech-language pathologist
Patient needs		
Setting		
Regulations		
Collaborators		

Looking at the shared responsibilities and complementary responsibilities that you listed above, what drivers will determine how you collaborate to perform these professional activities? Think about patient needs, setting, regulations, and collaborators.

As described in the medication reconciliation example above, policies can be important for defining roles and responsibilities. However, policies take time to write and approve and are hard to change once they are enacted. How might you go about this process of writing a policy that defines roles and responsibilities for a complex healthcare task? What factors would you want to consider, and how would you approach the process of crafting and implementing the policy?

Further Reading

The benefit of using pharmacists to manage chronic disease has been demonstrated in a number of publications. The Asheville Project is a famous example. One article about this program and its outcomes for patients with diabetes is by Carole Cranor and colleagues, titled "The Asheville Project: Long-Term Clinical and Economic Outcomes of a Community Pharmacy Diabetes Care Program," in *The Journal of the American Pharmacists Association*, 2003.

Similar work has been done with hypertension. An example is by Barry Carter and colleagues, "A Cluster Randomized Trial to Evaluate Physician/Pharmacist Collaboration to Improve Blood Pressure Control," in *The Journal of Clinical Hypertension*, 2008.

Medication reconciliation is a challenging clinical activity. There are several review articles about medication reconciliation. I like Elin Lehnbom and colleagues' article, "Impact of Medication Reconciliation and Review on Clinical Outcomes," in *The Annals of Pharmacotherapy*, 2014, because it shows how complicated this area is, how common this problem is, and how little we know about how to do medication reconciliation well.

SECTION 3

The Structures of Interprofessional Practice

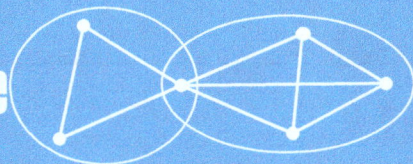

CHAPTER 4

Types of Work

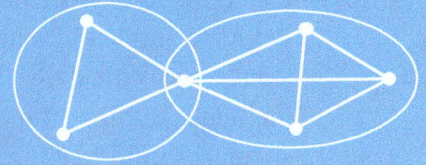

We've looked at the people side of healthcare by examining professions, scopes of practice, roles, and responsibilities. Now, let's look at the process of doing our work and how collaboration helps us work better. In this chapter, we will define four types of work to structure our thinking about collaboration. By the end of this chapter, you will be able to:

▸ differentiate four different types of work,
▸ discuss the implications of each type of work for collaboration, and
▸ describe how the four different types of work can go wrong.

Initial Reflection Questions

Think about the activities that you participate in. Some might be related to work or school, while others might occur during time you spend with your friends or while you're doing chores around the house. Name some activities that meet the following characteristics:

Routine activities that you can do individually without much thought. We will label these types of activities as *simple work*.

Routine activities during which you work in parallel with others but don't require much ongoing interaction. We will label these types of activities as *complicated work*.

Nonroutine activities that require both ongoing interaction with others. We will label these types of activities as *complex work*.

Simple Work

Simple work is routine. Doing the work correctly invariably leads to a good result. Simple work does not require additional expertise; it is clear how to approach this work. Examples of activities that count as simple work in daily life for most people include washing the dishes, tying their shoelaces, and making a sandwich.

Typical training to become a healthcare professional prepares us to do the simple work of our standard professional activities. Some examples of simple work in healthcare include completing routine patient assessments, analyzing data from assessments, or conducting straightforward tests or other procedures. Simple work is usually done individually. Uncertainty is low, and conflict is unlikely.

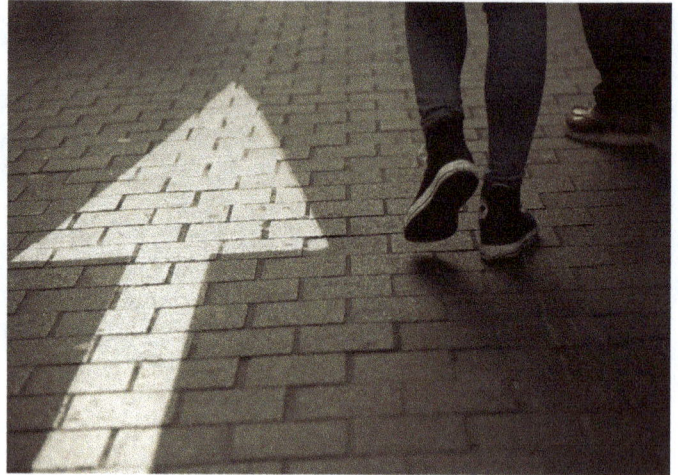

However, simple work is not risk-free. Errors can lead to problems including patient harm. Errors are usually not due to uncertainty or ignorance but rather other factors. Complacency or lack of attention to detail can be a source of error. Simple work can be mind-numbing. Someone not focused on the job could overlook a key piece of information or skip an important step, such as not taking an alcohol use history from a patient or failing to carefully review old records. Technical mistakes can also happen, such as an error during a procedure.

The literature on diagnostic error in healthcare demonstrates the challenges of simple work. The most common cause of an error in diagnosis is called *premature closure*. Premature closure is when a clinician decides on a diagnosis too soon and then disregards or fails to identify information that goes against that diagnosis. In this case, clinicians think they are doing simple work when in fact they are dealing with a more challenging case and have failed to make the correct diagnosis (see sidebar).

Simple work in healthcare may feel easy, but it requires persistence and attention to detail. Our professional activities can seem rote and ritualistic, but we need to be alert and recognize when seemingly simple work is not so simple after all.

A Not-so-Simple Case of Pneumonia

When I was newly in practice, we were taking care of a young man admitted to the hospital with pneumonia. He was fairly sick when he was admitted, with a high fever and an elevated white blood cell count. We started him on antibiotics. I was sure he would be better in a couple of days. This seemed like a simple case of pneumonia.

After three days, he was worse. His fever continued, and his white cell count was even higher. His chest X-ray showed that the pneumonia was expanding. I wondered if I was wrong about his diagnosis, so I called the pulmonologists (lung doctors) to see him and evaluate him for a bronchoscopy, a procedure in which you put a scope through the mouth and into the airways, look at the lungs, and take samples for laboratory analysis. They agreed to perform the bronchoscopy, in part because it was Friday and they did not want to leave things unresolved over the weekend.

During the bronchoscopy, the patient's breathing worsened, to the point that he required a breathing tube (intubation) and transfer to the ICU. The next day, the sample from the bronchoscopy revealed that he had blastomycosis, a fungus that can cause unusual cases of pneumonia. Treating this fungus requires different antibiotics (antifungals) than we usually use. Once he was started on the antifungal medication in the ICU, he quickly improved. About a week later, I sent him home from the hospital.

Fortunately, I kept an open mind to other possibilities. If I had not, this 'simple' case could have been fatal.

Complicated Work

Like simple work, complicated work is routine. However, complicated work requires additional expertise and collaboration between individuals. Even though it takes additional expertise to reach the optimal result, the best approach is clear and should be guided by evidence and best practices. If that approach is implemented, the outcome will be positive. However, additional effort is required with complicated work to *coordinate* the expertise and activities of different individuals. Much of the work is done in parallel, and people need to be aware of each other's roles and responsibilities. Examples of complicated work might be building a house, organizing a large event, or sailing a boat. The important point is that you usually can't do these things by yourself.

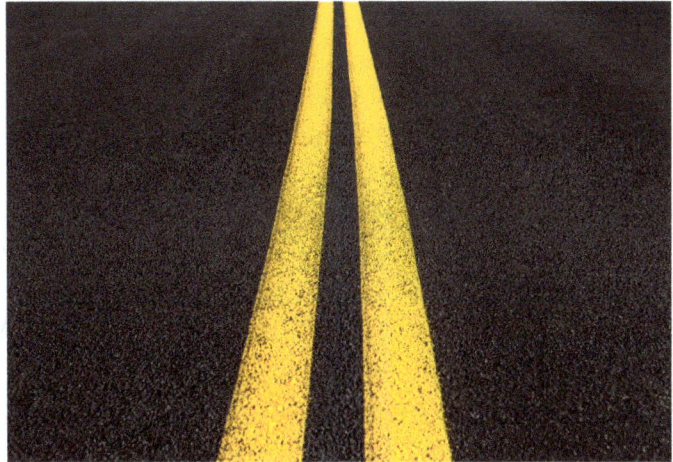

© turtix/Shutterstock.com

Complicated work is our typical way of working in healthcare. Any time different expertise is needed to care for a patient—which is almost always—practitioners are engaging in complicated work. Patients' individual health conditions drive the needed expertise and the interactions between the practitioners caring for patients. Certain individuals may emerge as leaders.

Complicated work brings different challenges than simple work does. The coordination between healthcare professionals takes effort. If that coordination falters, errors can happen, and patients may receive suboptimal care or even be harmed. In addition, the facility's systems may or may not be set up to support the needed coordination for complicated work.

At my hospital, for example, I can get almost any help I need for my patients to complete the complicated work of their care—unless it's a weekend. Then, my options for help are more limited. Fewer people are around, and those people have expanded responsibilities. This is true across professions. The systems is better staffed to tackle complicated problems on weekdays. Sometimes, I decide whether to put in the effort to engage in complicated work on the weekend or just wait until Monday, when there will be more people around to make the complicated work easier.

The key to complicated work in healthcare is learning how to work within the system to coordinate care. Sometimes these coordination processes are explicitly established or taught. For example, at my hospital, we have a paging process through which nurses communicate issues to covering physicians. Depending on the level of concern around the issue, the nurse chooses an approach to paging, from something of little concern ("FYI . . .") to a direct request for a significant concern ("Need you at bedside ASAP.").

More commonly, practitioners must figure out the coordination process through trial and error or word of mouth. Coordination of complicated work often depends more on the relationships between healthcare professionals and the culture of the setting. We will discuss these issues in much greater detail, but for now, recognize that complicated work is about coordinating across healthcare professionals to help a patient.

Complex Work

Complex work is where collaboration gets especially challenging. Complex work is uncertain and unpredictable. Like complicated work, complex work almost always involves additional expertise, but unlike complicated work, the best approach remains uncertain. There is no obvious solution to achieve the best outcome. Experts may disagree, and there may be conflict. Examples of complex work include raising a child, decorating a house, and educating people for future careers.

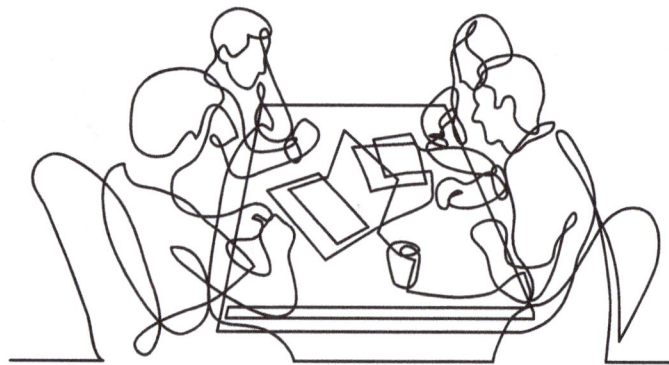

© one line man/Shutterstock.com

In healthcare, complex work is less frequent than complicated work, but it takes up more time and resources. Because complex work has less clarity around the best course of action, the decision-making is more challenging. It can be exhausting and stressful. Patient preferences, which are important in all types of healthcare work, take on more weight because there are a number of possible courses of action. Think about that for a moment: as decision-making becomes more challenging, patients, rather than experts, play a more critical role in making those decisions.

Consider the decision to continue or cease cancer treatment. Unfortunately, millions of people each year decide whether to receive chemotherapy or not. No one wants to die from cancer. Nor does anyone want to needlessly experience the side effects of chemotherapy. Physicians, nurses, chaplains, and others can advise the patient and his or her family, but the patient must be at the center of grappling with that decision.

Complex work is the hardest work in healthcare. It's messy and uncertain. It requires open communication among practitioners, patients, and families. It can be emotionally charged, causing people—both patients and practitioners—to scream or cry.

It can also be some of the most fulfilling work in healthcare. Doing complex work well requires wisdom, empathy, and compassion. The reason people fail at complex work is that they do not engage in it fully. It requires us to be our best selves, both in our work and collaboratively.

We'll talk more about how to do complex work in the rest of the book, but, for now, think of complex work as work that requires collaboration to figure out how to best navigate uncertainty.

Chaotic Work

You probably noticed that the initial reflection questions only covered the first three types of work. The final type of work, chaotic work, is far less common. Chaotic work is unpredictable and disordered. It is unclear what you should do when engaged with chaotic work. Chaotic work can be creative and is useful in the arts. Sometimes, businesses engage in chaotic work as a way of stimulating innovation, but it can lack purpose and be unproductive.

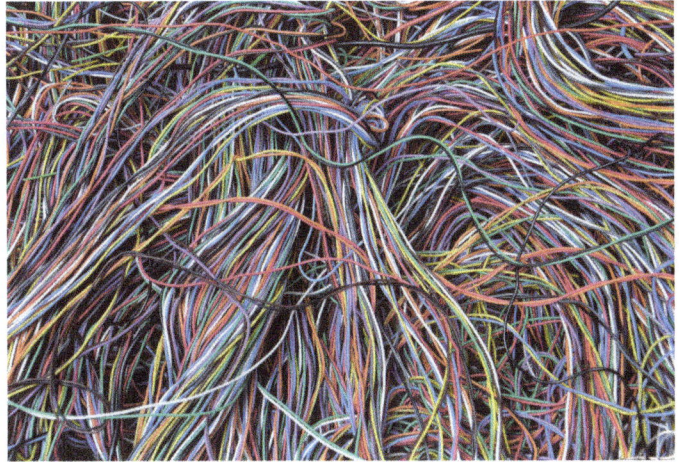

© Flegere/Shutterstock.com

Chaotic work is rare in healthcare because we always have the clear goal of helping patients. In addition, we work in systems that are planned out, supplied with resources, have processes for communication, and have defined roles and responsibilities for practitioners. But, sometimes, the system breaks down.

An example of chaotic work in healthcare is responding to a medical emergency outside of a care facility, where you are thrust into the role of healthcare practitioner without any of the usual resources around you. I once came to the aid of a man who was in cardiac arrest at a restaurant. I was terrified: I had no idea what help was around me or what was going to happen from one moment to the next. But I had been trained in CPR and advanced life support and, fortunately, a nurse practitioner and a nurse also responded to his family's call for help. We started CPR, and soon the EMTs arrived, defibrillated his heart, got his heart beating again, and whisked him off to the hospital. Note what happened: chaotic work turned into complicated work when a collaborating team arrived. And the man survived. He and I met up at that same restaurant a couple of months later.

The main point about chaotic work is that it generally does not last long in healthcare. We are well trained, and we know how to find the resources and create the structure we need to help our patients. But it's important to recognize when you're in chaos and figure out how to move forward out of it.

Application Questions

Thinking about your current or future career, list some activities that you will frequently engage in that fall into each of these categories:

Simple work:

Complicated work:

Complex work:

Final Reflection Questions

The biggest risks with simple work are making errors due to cutting corners and not recognizing that the work is not simple. What approaches can you use in your current or future work to avoid these risks?

The biggest risk with complicated work is failure of coordination. What are some of the reasons why coordination might fail? How might you prevent these failures?

Complex work requires more effort than either simple or complicated work. How does this additional effort affect how you should approach complex work to ensure that you and your colleagues are as successful as possible?

Chaotic work is often the most challenging type of work to identify. Can you think of any examples?

Further Reading

The types of work presented in this chapter reflect an adapted and simplified version of the Cynefin framework, first published in "A Leader's Framework for Decision Making," a November 2007 article in the *Harvard Business Review*. This framework has been applied to healthcare in a number of articles. Some good examples to start with include:

- "Complexity and Health—Yesterday's Traditions, Tomorrow's Future" by Joachim Sturmberg and Carmel Martin in the *Journal of Evaluation in Clinical Practice* (June 2009).

- "Notes From a Small Island: Researching Organisational Behaviour in Healthcare From a UK Perspective" by Annabelle Mark in the *Journal of Organizational Behavior* (November 2006).

CHAPTER 5

Structure of Groups

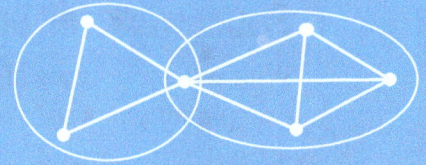

Now that we've talked about professions and types of work, it is finally time to look at how various professions interact during interprofessional practice. The different ways in which groups collaborate will be the foundation for the rest of this book. By the end of this chapter, you should be able to:

▸ compare and contrast teamwork, coordination, and networking;
▸ give examples of teamwork, coordination, and networking in healthcare;
▸ identify how each group structure intersects with the different types of work.

Initial Reflection Questions

Think about a time when you planned something outside of work with a group of people. It could be a social event, a vacation, or something else. How did you work together to plan the event? How much of the planning was done face-to-face versus over the phone or by other means?

How much of the planning was done with everyone working at the same time (synchronously) versus at separate times (asynchronously)?

What processes and technology did you use to support the planning process?

Why did you approach planning in that fashion? What were the advantages and disadvantages of your approach?

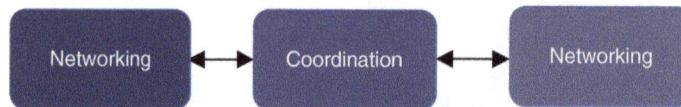

Figure 5.1 Spectrum of Group Collaboration. Source: Alan Dow.

Framework for Group Collaboration

Within the four types of work—simple, complicated, complex, and chaotic—how do groups of health-care practitioners collaborate with one another to improve health outcomes? Let's define a framework for different forms of group collaboration (see Figure 5.1) to help us think through the ways that groups can collaborate. This framework is a spectrum with teamwork, the most synchronous and tightly knit form of collaboration, at one end and networking, the most asynchronous and loosest form of collaboration, at the other end. Let's look at each form of group collaboration individually.

Teamwork

When you think of collaboration, you likely first think of *teamwork* (Figure 5.2). Teams are familiar to us from sports and other contexts. But let's take a moment to examine the specific definition we'll be using for a team.

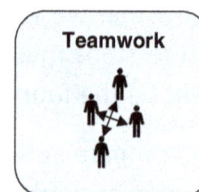

Figure 5.2 An Interdependent, Closely Working Team. Source: Alan Dow.

- **Teams are groups of people with complementary skills working toward a single goal.** So far, that sounds like our interprofessional healthcare groups, which combine our profession-specific abilities to work together toward the goal of improving patients' health.
- **Teams are interdependent.** This also sounds like healthcare based on our understanding of complicated and complex work. We depend on each other to do these types of work.
- **Teams share authority, accountability, responsibility, and an understanding of the work.** Here's where we falter as teams in healthcare. Despite our interdependence, we often don't have the opportunity to truly become a team. We usually don't have structures to help us share authority and accountability. While we share responsibilities, we sometimes don't share an understanding of the work we're doing, especially when we are working in different places or at different times. In addition, we may be evaluated and reimbursed for services in different ways, so our incentives are not aligned.

Challenges to Teamwork: A Case Study

A group of colleagues and I studied the array of healthcare practitioners involved in the care of cancer patients during the first 60 days after their diagnosis with cancer. What we found shocked us.

First, the number of practitioners involved in each patient's care was astounding. A typical patient had 117 practitioners involved in her care. One patient had 440 practitioners! You can imagine trying to get 117 practitioners on the same page. Forming a true team with that many members would be impossible.

Second, we could not easily predict which practitioners would be involved in each patient's care. Care was complex. Patients' needs changed as they developed other problems or as their practitioners changed the course of their treatment. That's a good thing—it's patient-centered—but it makes predicting whether a healthcare practitioner would be involved with a patient challenging. Even trying to form a team with a subgroup of practitioners would be a challenge.

Groups of practitioners in cancer care are too big and too complex for teamwork. We need a different approach.

There are two ways to think about fixing the teamwork problems in healthcare. One is by increasing and improving teamwork. This is an important goal, but it is often costly, and often, downright impossible (see sidebar). So, let's strive for better teamwork where we can and look to the second way to fix the teamwork problem: by getting better at other forms of group collaboration. Both ideas are themes of this book.

Still, we have some good examples of teamwork in healthcare: groups of practitioners in the operating room, well-functioning primary care practices, and some rehabilitation groups, to name a few. Yet, most collaboration is not well-integrated teamwork. This is not the fault of the practitioners; rather, the system itself is big and complex, and patients have unique individual needs that span multiple healthcare professionals.

Yes, we need great teams, but I generally use the term *group* rather than *team* throughout this book because teams are something special, and we need to recognize them as aspirational rather than standard in healthcare.

Coordination

A form of group collaboration that is looser than teamwork is *coordination* (Figure 5.3). When we discussed the types of work in the last chapter, specifically complicated work, we hinted at the importance of coordination. For now, I want you to be able to contrast coordination with teamwork.

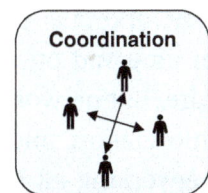

Figure 5.3 A More Diffuse Group Working in Coordination. Source: Alan Dow.

During coordination, practitioners have opportunities for face-to-face interaction and integrated planning like they do in teamwork, but they generally work separately. Coordination is the staple of complicated work; individuals work in parallel, but they are aware of each other's work and available to assist each other. The line between teamwork and coordination can be blurry, but the difference is important because of the implications for how collaboration works.

Think about a typical group of healthcare practitioners in an inpatient unit, clinic, or rehabilitation setting. The group may meet daily or weekly to talk about what patients they have and how the work has been going. There is a shared understanding between them of the approach to work and each practitioner's roles and responsibilities, even if this understanding is not explicitly stated. But, in contrast to a team, most of their patient care activities are done individually, and the practitioners are less interdependent. The group may have less of a shared identity. While the group could form into a team (around a specific project or if a patient's condition demands teamwork), generally these practitioners are working on their own.

Coordination is essential for the best care. It requires less time from healthcare professionals and costs less to the overall system. But it increases the chance of miscommunication, exclusion of a valuable perspective, or another error. Overall, coordination is one of the key ways we collaborate in healthcare, and we will explore this process in greater depth in Chapter 8.

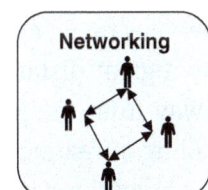

Figure 5.4 A Network Within Which Not All Group Members Are Directly Connected. Source: Alan Dow.

Networking

The loosest form of group collaboration in our framework is *networking* (Figure 5.4). In networking, practitioners can work at different times (asynchronously) and even in different places (non-co-located). A common example is a patient who receives health services from both a primary care office and a community pharmacy. After the practitioners in the primary care office have made a diagnosis, prescribed a treatment, and communicated this prescription to the patient and the pharmacy, the practitioners in the pharmacy fill the prescription and dispense the medication to the patient. Practitioners in both settings share some of the same professional activities, such as counseling the patient. Yet, the practitioners have not communicated with each other or developed a shared model for the patient's care.

During networking, collaboration is occurring, but the opportunities for face-to-face interaction are few. Work is not shared through direct interaction. Rather, the structure of the system defines how work is shared. For example, scope of practice determines roles, responsibilities, and expectations for how different professionals interact as they fulfill those roles and responsibilities. Likewise, available technological tools like electronic health records, phone calls, and faxes define the interactions within a network.

The border between networking and other types of collaboration is porous. Networks can shift into coordination or teamwork if needed. For example, if the pharmacist calls the primary care practitioner to ask questions related to the prescription, those practitioners are now engaging in coordination or perhaps even teamwork.

Networking is common in healthcare. Of the types of collaboration, it requires the least investment of time and other resources. In many ways, it is the standard state of practice for much of healthcare. But networking can easily lead to error. There are more chances for miscommunication, missed information, and mistakes arising from a lack of a shared understanding of the work. We engage in networking all the time, and it's good for routine, low-risk work, but you would never attempt an organ transplant via networking.

Integrating Types of Work and Types of Collaboration

Let's start with simple work. As you know, simple work can usually be done by an individual; you don't need a group of healthcare practitioners. Yet, nothing in healthcare is done in isolation. We are always working in groups, even when the collaboration is "loose," meaning that the practitioners are only weakly associated with each other. When you are doing simple work, your role as a collaborator is to recognize how your work might interface with the simple work of other practitioners via coordination or networking. How does your piece of the puzzle fit into the larger picture? Who else is also working to help this patient?

This means that your simple work doesn't stand alone; it is always part of a larger pattern of complicated work. Multiple practitioners are doing their own pieces of simple work to accomplish the goal of improving a patient's health. These individual pieces of simple work might be occurring simultaneously or asynchronously. They might be occurring in the same location, or they might be separated by a great distance. Think about the laboratory technician analyzing a sample in a lab many miles away from the patient in the hospital. Or the athletic trainer on the sideline of a game who is providing a treatment based on the recommendations of a physical therapist. Or the dentist in an office examining a patient who receives primary health services in a different location.

Some of this complicated work may be done through coordination, while other parts may be done through networking. Your responsibility is to recognize what type or types of collaboration you are taking part in and how you can enhance those types of collaboration. That's where we are headed in the rest of the book.

What about complex and chaotic work? As I described in the last chapter, chaotic work usually quickly evolves into another type of work, most commonly complex or complicated work. Complex work also shares this feature: because it is resource-intensive, hard work, it tends to evolve into less intensive work.

However, while we would never choose chaotic work, we sometimes need complex work to best meet our patients' needs. Because the best approach is uncertain in complex work, we need to get together in a more intensive form of collaboration, usually teamwork, to determine the best path forward. Sometimes, coordination may the best we can do, but think of complex work as the motivation driving the necessity for teamwork. We need the best of all of us to navigate the complexity of healthcare.

Multi-Team Systems

One description of interprofessional practice that delineates the intricacies of collaboration in healthcare is a *multi-team system*. A multi-team system is a network of teams (for the moment, let's leave out coordination as an intermediary step). In a multi-team system, healthcare practitioners each work as part of a team, and each team is part of a network of other teams. Let me give you an example.

Think about an individual who has been in a car accident. A group consisting of paramedics, police officers, and firefighters arrives at the scene to provide aid. These individuals work collaboratively to assist the victim. Leadership is decided based on the issues at hand; firefighters ensure safety and usually have the most authority unless there is an issue with violence or crime over which the police have authority. The paramedics have the least authority over the scene but the most authority over the health needs of the victim.

Once the paramedics have assessed and provided initial treatment to the victim, they transport the victim to an emergency department. During the trip, the paramedics engage in networking or coordination activities, notifying the practitioners in the emergency department of their estimated arrival, giving the status of the victim, and communicating any anticipated needs. When the paramedics arrive with the victim at the emergency department, care is handed over to the practitioners there.

Now, a new group of nurses, physicians, technicians, and others collaborates to assess and provide further treatment to the patient. Membership in this group evolves based on the patient's needs. Depending on the victim's needs, these practitioners may incorporate additional individuals into the group, perhaps an orthopedist for a broken bone or a radiology technician to perform X-rays.

At some point, the victim will be ready to leave the emergency department. He may be transferred to a hospital unit for further inpatient care by another group of nurses, doctors, pharmacists, and others. Or he may be discharged home to be cared for by a group of outpatient practitioners.

The key point of this example is to see the different structures of teamwork, networking, and coordination and how they interact and adapt. Four groups—the on-scene emergency response professionals, the emergency department practitioners, the inpatient practitioners, and the outpatient practitioners—may all have responsibility for the patient at some point. Collaboration occurs not only within these groups but also between these groups through coordination and networking.

Healthcare practitioners often work within all three types of groups, and being aware of how these structures shape your work and the effectiveness of your work is critical. In addition, recognizing how you and your patients move between these structures is an essential ability for ensuring that your patients have the best possible outcomes.

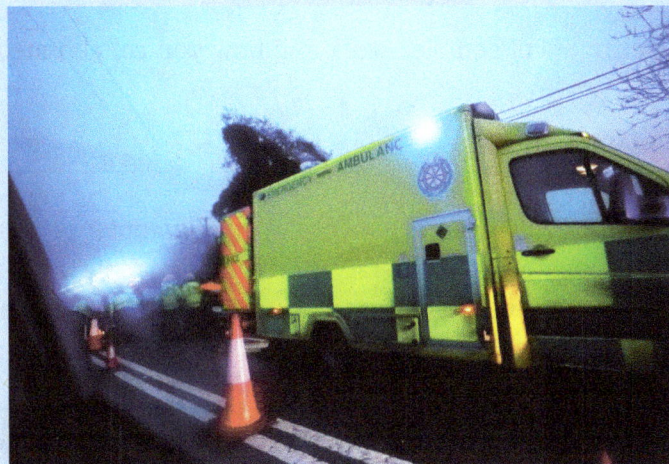

Application Questions

Thinking about your life so far, give an example of when you engaged in each of the following types of work and the role of collaboration in completing various activities as part of that work. While health-related examples are ideal, you can also provide examples from schoolwork or other activities.

An example of primarily simple work and any ways that collaboration related to this work:

An example of complicated work and how you collaborated with others:

An example of complex work and how you collaborated with others:

Let's also consider your experience with different types of collaboration. Give an example for each and describe a way that you interacted with other people in the group. Again, try to think of health-related examples, but you can pull from educational or personal experiences, if need be.

An example of teamwork and how you interacted with other team members:

An example of coordination and how you interacted with other team members:

An example of networking and how you interacted with other team members:

While I have presented collaboration as having three distinct types—teamwork, coordination, and networking—these types exist along a spectrum with indistinct borders. What do you see as the key differences among these three different types of collaboration? How and why are these differences important to providing health services?

Final Reflection Questions

Thinking about your current or future practice as a healthcare practitioner, describe an example of a group of which you might be a member. What is a situation that could be described as complex work requiring closer collaboration among the group members? How might group members identify that this situation is complex and recognize the need for greater collaboration among group members?

Can you think of some current examples where the type of collaboration occurring does not meet the needs of patients? Why not?

Further Reading

The different types of interprofessional practice described here stem from the work of Scott Reeves and others in the book *Interprofessional Teamwork for Health and Social Care* (Wiley-Blackwell, 2010). A recent publication that expanded on this work is "Teamwork, Collaboration, Coordination, and Networking: Why We Need to Distinguish Between Different Types of Interprofessional Practice" by Scott Reeves, Andreas Xyrichis, and Merrick Zwarenstein in the *Journal of Interprofessional Care* (November 2017). Despite this area's fundamental importance to interprofessional practice, it is still emerging and evolving; I have endeavored to provide a simple and clear distillation of this literature to allow a basic understanding of the concepts. Read more if you have interest.

CHAPTER 6

Drivers of Collaboration

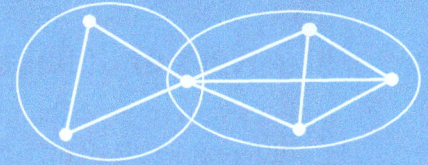

A theme of this book is the dynamic nature of collaboration. Patterns of collaboration shift over time, and understanding why and how these shifts happen provides a foundation for being a more effective healthcare practitioner as conditions change. At the end of the chapter on roles and responsibilities, we looked at several drivers of an individual's professional responsibilities. In this chapter, we will expand those ideas to collaboration. Looking at these drivers shape collaboration will prepare us over the next two chapters to examine groups and how they evolve and collaborate. By the end of this chapter, you will be able to:

▸ identify the patient, group, organizational, and societal drivers that shape collaboration;

▸ explain how those different drivers affect patient outcomes; and

▸ describe how to influence these drivers to enhance collaboration.

Initial Reflection Questions

Think of a time when you were involved in supporting someone's health. Providing direct care to a patient would be the best example, but if you are new to healthcare, you can think of a time when you had a family member who needed your support. Think about which healthcare practitioners collaborated with you to support this person's health and how you all interacted.

What factors at the level of the <u>patient</u> shaped that collaboration? Think about factors like the health condition or diagnosis, social support from friends and family, or other factors specific to the patient's background.

What factors at the level of the <u>group of healthcare practitioners</u> shaped collaboration? Think about the healthcare practitioners involved in the patient's care and how they interacted.

What factors at the level of the <u>organization</u> shaped collaboration? Think about the setting, technology, and aspects of the place where care was delivered beyond the group of healthcare practitioners who were involved. Don't forget to consider organizational culture as we described it in chapter 3.

What factors at the level of <u>society</u> shaped collaboration? Think about laws, regulations, insurance, and broad cultural factors outside of the healthcare setting.

Drivers of Collaboration at Different Levels

Let's start by describing a framework for thinking about the different levels of drivers of collaboration (see Figure 6.1). At the center of the framework is the patient, including the patient's family and his or her life beyond this immediate healthcare situation. The next level includes group drivers, such as which professions are collaborating and what process they use for collaboration. The third level represents organizational drivers. An example is the resources the organization provides for care such as people, technology, facilities, equipment, and anything else that supports delivering health services. Finally, the outermost level includes societal drivers including laws, policies, and the broader societal culture.

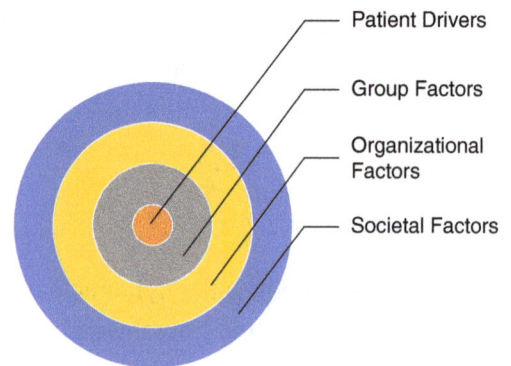

Figure 6.1 Different Levels of Drivers of Collaboration. Source: Alan Dow.

Even though I am describing these levels as distinct, the borders between levels are not necessarily clean. For example, educational policy, a societal driver, influences the level of education that a patient might have attained, which is a patient factor. Keep in mind I am oversimplifying the relationship between these levels for the sake of learning about what they are and how they influence collaboration.

Patient Drivers

Patient drivers encompass the patient's entire life! The patient's presenting health need tends to be the driver at this level that gets most of the attention. Patients seek health care for routine follow-up, screening and health promotion, rehabilitation, acute health needs, and other reasons. As interprofessional collaborators, our responsibilities include identifying who else, if anyone, needs to be involved to meet that presenting health need. If patients require more help than you can provide alone, it is up to you to lead the process of expanding collaboration. If you decide that this patient doesn't need help from any other practitioner, or you fail to ask the question, you might miss an opportunity to better help the patient.

Of course, none of us is defined by only one issue. Patient drivers also include other health conditions that might influence the main health issue. These are the areas you commonly touch on when taking a health history: acute and chronic diagnoses, fertility history and plans, and substance use patterns, for example. We ask those questions for a reason. Because you are a conscientious practitioner, you will regularly discover other health conditions that interact with a patient's primary health need. As you identify these additional patient drivers, you may need to add collaborators to fully address them.

Patient drivers also include areas beyond health conditions, the so-called social determinants of health. Examples include family structure, educational status, income level, housing, race, ethnicity, gender, sexual orientation, and other factors. Social determinants of health can have positive or negative effects; for example, married people have a better prognosis after a cancer diagnosis than people who are single or divorced. Here again, your job is to identify these issues and recognize how they should shape collaborative care for patients. Someone with more barriers to health may need more support—for example, more time spent on patient education—and your group needs to determine who will provide that support and how it will be provided.

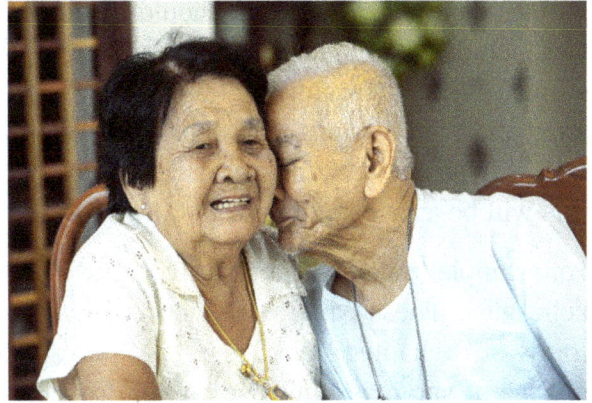
© WitthayaP/Shutterstock.com

Group Drivers

In contrast to patient drivers of collaboration, group drivers of collaboration are something you can directly influence as a healthcare practitioner. Group drivers are not always obvious. Let's group them as either explicit or hidden. *Explicit factors* are readily apparent to someone who engages with a group, while *hidden factors* are less obvious. Both define local culture and how we collaborate, but recognizing the difference is important.

Explicit factors include who is in the group, what defined responsibilities each person has, and how interactions between those individuals are formalized. Often, explicit factors are systematized as procedures, policies, or scopes of practice (see sidebar) that define how work should be done.

Responsibility vs. Expertise

Let's contrast responsibility and expertise. As we noted in chapter 3, *responsibility* is being accountable for an area, while *expertise* is specialized knowledge or skill in an area. Where we have overlap in expertise among individuals in a collaborative group, we need to define responsibility. Often it doesn't make sense for the most expert person to be responsible. Let me give you an example.

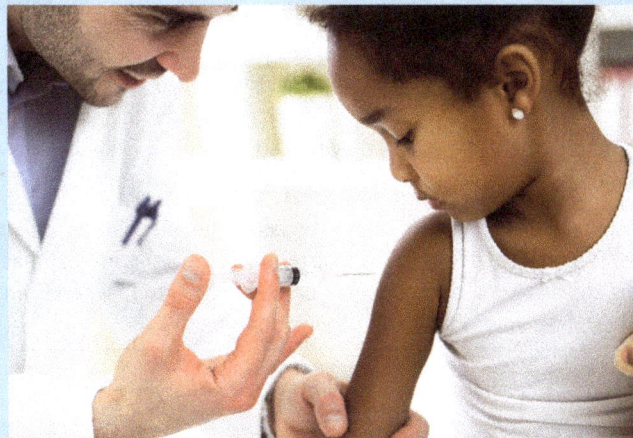
© didesign021/Shutterstock.com

Vaccination schedules are created by experts at organizations like the Centers for Disease Control and the World Health Organization. But the responsibility for administering vaccinations falls to frontline entities like primary care practices, pharmacies, and other community-facing organizations. Within these entities, the most expert practitioners are generally lousy at following algorithms like vaccine schedules. Their problem-solving skills are better applied to patients with undiagnosed health needs. They're trained to think through complex and dynamic situations rather than follow a standard protocol.

What works best to improve vaccination rates is to have a system where someone is responsible for ensuring that vaccines are given according to a schedule. This person, for example, a medical assistant, uses a protocol to screen patients for vaccination needs and to administer vaccinations within the guidelines of the protocol.

While you need experts to help create the protocol, you then need those experts to get out of the way and let someone else be responsible for implementation.

Rather than being how work should be done, hidden factors define how work is done. Hidden factors include what patterns of collaboration individuals have learned from prior work together, who is seen as a leader (regardless of what title or role each person has), and what stereotypes practitioners have about professions that shape collaboration (see sidebar). Hidden factors interact with explicit factors to shape work in a particular context, but the hidden factors are more influential. Hidden factors will be a theme of the rest of the book.

For example, we all like familiarity, and we often settle into a certain way of working with a group of colleagues. Those patterns are normal, and they help with sharing of responsibilities as we will see in the next chapter. Often, those ways of working are not written down or required, and they may change or vary over time. Next year, down the street, or around the corner, very similar work may be done very differently.

Professional Tribes

Becoming part of a profession means joining a professional tribe. Each profession has certain characteristics: for example, how members dress, what they commonly do, or how they interact with other healthcare practitioners. So, congratulations, welcome to your tribe.

Of course, being part of a tribe creates a problem. It inherently puts us in an "us vs. them" situation where we assess people as either part of or not part of our tribe. We forget that the characteristics of the tribe are merely stereotypes that, at best, are lazy shortcuts for understanding individuals and, at worst, are harmful to our relationships and our patient care.

In one study by Melissa Valentine and Amy Edmondson, assigning healthcare practitioners in the emergency department to specific roles rather than just having them shift roles within their professional scopes of practice had dramatic impacts on performance. The groups performed better, and patients left the emergency department much faster. But, there was a downside. The physicians felt that the assigned roles weakened the camaraderie within their profession. Under the new system, they missed their tribe! Because tribes are powerful, the idea has not spread quickly across emergency departments.

Becoming part of a tribe is normal; as part of the process of forming into groups, it's called *norming*, which we will discuss later. The challenge for us is to recognize our tribal nature and reach beyond our tribe to include others. We are all part of many tribes at work: our profession, unit, shift, age group, gender, and others. That's natural, but it can prevent us from being our best if we aren't mindful to expand our tribe.

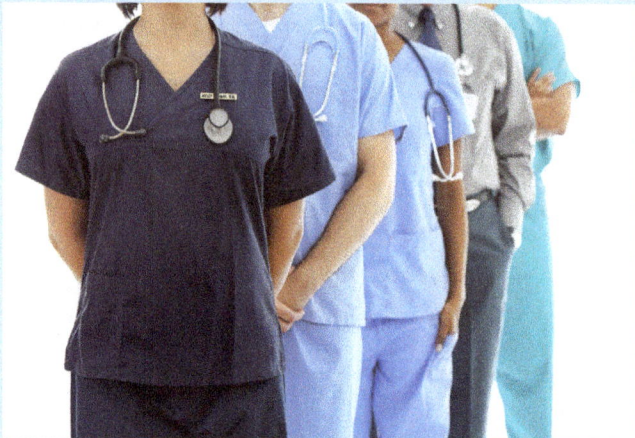

Hidden factors also demonstrate who we are. All of us like certain tasks or working with certain people better than others, and you can see that in how a group collaborates. Responsibilities are shaped based on personal preference and personality. Usually, that's not explicit.

Which brings us to your role with group drivers of collaboration. One of your most important responsibilities is to enhance interprofessional practice through group drivers. Usually this starts with hidden factors. Think about how you and your colleagues work and why. How could it be better? As you identify the impact of hidden factors, you may either want to make them explicit or change them via some explicit process like a new policy or protocol.

Where you work is a soup in which you, your patients, and your colleagues are all swimming. We bathe in the culture that is that soup, and it flavors our lives. The explicit factors are the components of that soup and when they enter the broth. Are they the right ingredients and the right amount for what your patients need? If not, can you change them? The hidden factors are how everything mingles together once it's in the pot. Are we collaborating in the best way to help our patients? Do all of us, including you and your colleagues, emerge from the soup better for swimming in it? Group drivers are the most direct way to change how you work. Pay attention to them.

Organizational Drivers

Organizational drivers and group drivers are interwoven. The decisions made by institutional leaders directly shape explicit group drivers. Examples include levels of staffing and professional roles defined by institutional policy. But let's look at a subtler example: the electronic health record.

Decisions about the electronic health record are a good example of how organizations impact both explicit and hidden factors that determine group collaboration. Impact on explicit factors includes decisions like who has what responsibilities in the electronic health record (see sidebar). But, that impact on explicit factors also shapes hidden factors like how information flows between professions.

For example, the notes of providers like physicians, nurse practitioners, physician's assistants, and dentists are often collected in the same folder. However, documentation from other practitioners such as nurses, respiratory therapists, and social workers might be excluded from this folder. The upside of this exclusion is that it limits the volume of information presented to each provider; information overload is a huge problem in healthcare and drives a lot of provider burnout. But the downsides are the potential exclusion of important information and reinforcement of traditional and outdated professional hierarchy. As a response to these downsides, many areas try to have interprofessional rounds to review information that is often overlooked in the electronic health record.

Allergies in the Electronic Health Record: Order or Documentation

In my health system's electronic health record, any licensed practitioner can update the allergy list. This seems like a good thing: collecting an allergy history is a straightforward, shared professional activity, and updating the list supports better communication and patient care. But there are naysayers.

The allergy list sometimes has errors. Most are mistakes in judgment. For example, an opiate medication might be entered as an allergy because it caused constipation, a known and common side effect of opiates but not truly an allergy. As another example, when a patient develops a rash thought to be due to a medication, some practitioners may enter all the medications that the patient is taking as an allergy. Later, the patient may not recall the details of a listed allergy, and prescribing becomes more difficult.

As a result, some practitioners have argued that the allergy list should be treated like a medication order and that updating it should be limited to prescribers like physicians. However, many practitioners—nurses and pharmacists, for example—have the expertise to update the allergy list. And, updating the allergy list can be life-saving, so we don't want to have to rely on just a couple professions to remember to do it. Oh, and one more thing—some of the errors in allergy lists were being made by prescribers.

For now, any licensed practitioner is still able to update the allergy list. But, it's worth recognizing that this is an area of conflict, and, as we will see in Chapter 11, you have to weigh the alternatives and their underlying values as you make decisions that shape professional responsibilities and the ways we collaborate.

Think of organizational drivers are choices. These choices may not be easy (and they may not be your choices to make). As we will see when we look at decision-making, all options, including the decision not to make a choice, can have downsides. Moreover, consequences that occur may not have been recognized and intended. As healthcare practitioners, our role is to help our organization make better choices by providing our perspective to inform decision-making, monitoring for consequences in our practice environment, and advocating for change when necessary.

Societal Drivers

While societal drivers are the broadest level, they often bring us back to the patient at the innermost level. Laws, policy, insurance, and economic considerations shape how we deliver care via organizational and group drivers. At the same time, societal drivers also shape our patients' lives through the social determinants of health. Let's quickly examine the latter area first.

Remember, social determinants can be good or bad—level of education can be a plus or minus, for example—and we interact with these social determinants every day as we consider patients' current health status and how we can help them be as healthy as possible. Usually, we cannot shape an individual's social determinants of health, though sometimes we can help connect them to services for issues like hunger or homelessness. But that does not mean that we are powerless.

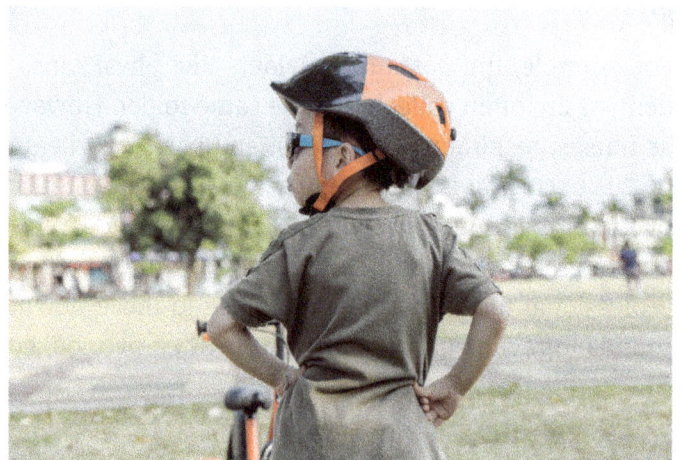

As healthcare practitioners, we know the stories of our patients and the challenges they face. We can be powerful advocates by providing them with a voice, particularly for individuals who are least able to advocate for themselves. While we can sometimes advocate for individual patients, our advocacy is more powerful for our community as a whole. We have the privilege of seeing how society affects our patients' health, and we should share that perspective to change society.

This advocacy links back to other connections between societal drivers and delivering care: laws, policies, payment structures, and others. Licensure and scope of practice are examples of how practice is shaped by laws. Societal drivers also shape how we collaborate; the biggest present-day example is how changes in payment models support increased collaboration (see sidebar).

New Ways of Paying for Healthcare

For decades in the United States, providers (such as physicians, nurse practitioners, physician's assistants, and dentists) have gotten paid by *fee-for-service*. Under fee-for-service, each service—an office visit, a daily visit in the hospital, a procedure—generates a bill that is reimbursed according to a fee schedule set by the insurer. More complicated activities get a higher fee: bypass surgery has a higher fee than an office visit.

Hospitals are paid in a similar fashion. They receive a certain amount for each day the patient is in the hospital or for each hospitalization. The amount is higher for more complex diagnoses.

Practitioners who are not providers are paid indirectly through these fees. A nurse in a clinic is paid a salary by the provider who initially received the payment from the insurer. Similarly, a nurse in a hospital is paid from the amount the hospital received for caring for the patient. Therapists, nutritionists, and other non-providers usually have the same arrangement.

Recognize the incentive here for providers and health systems: more care leads to more payment.

However, this approach is changing. Healthcare is expensive, and, to try to control spending, insurers are changing the incentives through approaches called alternative payment models. One type is an accountable care organization (ACO). Let's look at the incentives under an ACO and how they might change practice.

Under an ACO, instead of getting paid by the service, a local entity like a hospital gets paid a certain amount for a whole population, say $10,000 per person per year. If the entity can hold costs under $10,000 per person, it makes money, but if its costs exceed $10,000, the entity loses money.

Look at what this means for frontline practitioners. Now, the incentive is not to provide the most care; it is to control costs by providing the highest-value care. Keeping people away from expensive places in healthcare like hospitals and emergency departments becomes important. People with expertise in prevention and public health become increasingly valuable.

Under fee-for-service, a provider might be involved in a professional activity solely to generate a bill. But, under ACOs, if an activity does not require an expensive provider and can be more efficiently done by someone in another profession, then that other profession can now perform that activity without a financial penalty to anyone. An example is nurses being empowered to take larger roles in primary care. Individuals with expertise in communities, like public health practitioners, also become more important for shaping how care is delivered.

Application Questions

Thinking about your current practice or the role you would like to have in the future, answer the following questions:

What are or might be some common social determinants of health that affect your patients? How can these social determinants of health be either positive or negative? How can you affect these social determinants of health for an individual patient? For many patients?

What are or might be the group drivers of collaboration in your practice? Which are explicit, and which are hidden? How can you ensure that group drivers are supporting optimal collaboration?

What are or might be some organizational drivers of collaboration? What are mechanisms to advocate within your organization to improve collaboration? Can you identify any techniques used to support collaboration in the face of barriers to collaboration created by the organization?

Final Reflection Questions

Since patients should be at the center of care and drive the other levers of collaboration, how could patient factors be linked to the drivers of collaboration at other levels? Can you think of examples of how this might currently be happening?

What are the defining features of your professional tribe? Which of those features are generally true? Which are misconceptions? How do you differentiate yourself from the stereotypes of your professional tribe?

Alternative payment models like ACOs may change the responsibilities of different healthcare practitioners. What kind of changes might happen to your profession under these new ways of paying for healthcare?

Further Reading

Several authors have described different layers of levers when discussing interprofessional education. Although their layers differ from mine, these papers are worth reading to think about these different layers and the challenges at each layer.

- "Key Elements of Interprofessional Education. Part 2: Factors, Processes and Outcomes" by Ivy Oandasan and Scott Reeves in the *Journal of Interprofessional Care*, 2005, looks at micro, meso, and macro levels and each level's importance in interprofessional education.

- "Barriers and Enablers That Influence Sustainable Interprofessional Education: A Literature Review" by Tanya Lawlis, Judith Anson, and David Greenfield in the *Journal of Interprofessional Care*, 2014, reviews the literature to define the barriers to collaboration at each of these levels.

The impact of tribes in healthcare is outlined in "Teams, Tribes and Patient Safety: Overcoming Barriers to Effective Teamwork in Healthcare" by Jennifer Weller, Matt Boyd, and David Cumin in *The Postgraduate Medical Journal*, 2014.

In "Team Scaffolds: How Mesolevel Team Structures Enable Role-based Coordination in Temporary Groups" from *Organization Science* in 2015, Melissa Valentine and Amy Edmondson showed that having fixed roles (not just professions) improved team performance. But, physicians didn't like the intervention even though it improved performance because it broke up the physician tribe.

There are many resources that can help you learn more about alternative payment models like accountable care organizations. One place to start is the video and accompanying text published by Kaiser Health News at https://khn.org/news/aco-accountable-care-organization-faq/.

CHAPTER 7

Group Evolution

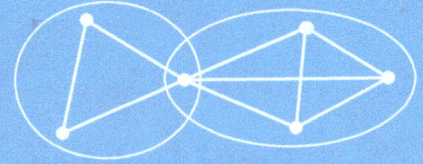

We've talked about the different types of collaboration, some drivers of collaboration at different levels within the healthcare system, and the ways these drivers affect the roles and responsibilities of healthcare practitioners. Collaboration evolves as healthcare practitioners transition into and between different groups. This chapter presents a common framework for the evolution of groups. This framework describes how groups turn into teams as their members become more interdependent and develop a shared approach to work. Understanding this framework helps identify why groups in healthcare find it especially challenging to form teams and how we can work toward better collaboration despite these challenges. By the end of this chapter, you should be able to:

▸ describe the five stages of group evolution,
▸ identify the challenges to collaboration in healthcare at each stage of group evolution, and
▸ recognize that practitioners belong to many groups at different stages of evolution and that optimal collaboration requires different approaches at each stage.

Initial Reflection

Think about a time when you joined a new group. The best example to consider would be a group related to healthcare, but if you haven't been involved in such a group yet, another experience is fine.

Describe how you became part of the group. Were you selected to be part of the group, or did you independently decide that you wanted to join the group? Was there a formal process of joining the group?

What was it like when you first joined the group? What challenges, if any, did you encounter being accepted by the group? How did you become a valuable member of the group?

How did your involvement in the group change over time? Does your involvement with the group continue? Has it ended? If so, how or why? Were there any events that marked a change in your role or an ending?

Group Evolution

Groups have a lifecycle. They are born, grow, and mature. Groups also sometimes dissolve, which is not necessarily a bad thing.

Healthcare practitioners belong to multiple co-existing groups. These multiple groups may be at multiple places in their lifecycles. How and if groups mature is shaped by the drivers of collaboration described in the last chapter.

The most mature form of a group is a *team*, characterized by members' interdependence and a shared understanding of how to approach the group's activities. The best teams, like a championship sports team, have gained an intuitive sense of how to work together.

This chapter introduces a framework to understand the lifecycle of a group. This framework was originally created by psychologist Bruce Tuckman beginning in the 1960s. He described five stages of group development: forming, storming, norming, performing, and adjourning (Figure 7.1). These stages will be the basis of this chapter. Understanding a group's stage of evolution helps members recognize how they can best collaborate within that group and possibly help the group mature to a more advanced stage.

Forming

Forming is the process of people coming together as a group. Because forming sets the foundation for how group members interact, it is a critical step in group evolution. And it is the most challenging stage in group development in healthcare.

Consider, for a moment, groups outside of healthcare. These groups are usually formed to focus on a particular project or set of tasks. Typically, members are selected through a careful hiring or selection process overseen by supervisors. Membership in the group is usually stable, meaning it rarely changes. When members are added, it is done deliberately. This type of project-based, intentional, stable group is called a work team, and it's a descriptive label—these groups usually meet our definition of interdependent teamwork.

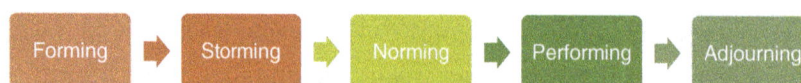

Forming ➡ Storming ➡ Norming ➡ Performing ➡ Adjourning

Figure 7.1 Tuckman's Stages of Group Development. Source: Alan Dow based on the work of Bruce Tuckman.

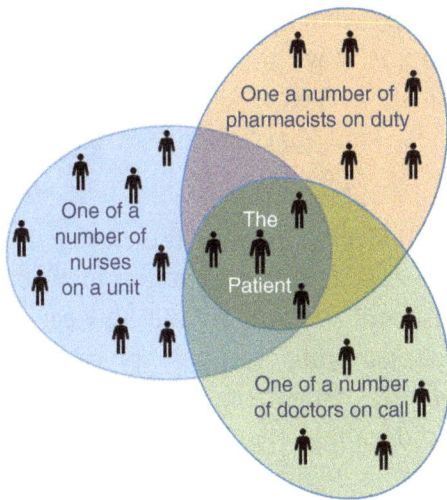

Figure 7.2 An Example of How a Patient May Have Nurses, Pharmacists, and Doctors Drawn from a Pool of People in Each Profession. Note the close working relationships of the most central practitioners. Source: Alan Dow.

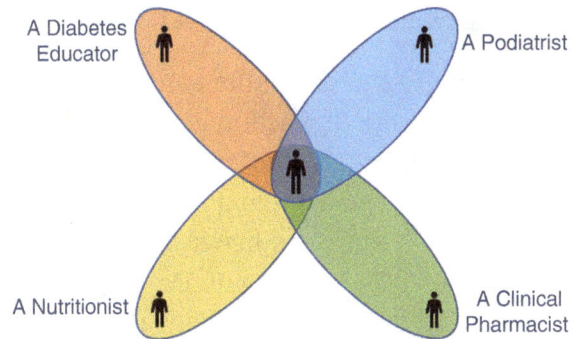

Figure 7.3 A Group of Healthcare Practitioners Caring for a Patient with Diabetes as a Network. They are not closely aligned and collaboration is more challenging. Source: Alan Dow.

Contrast this approach with what happens in healthcare group formation. In healthcare, group membership is often fluid, and that creates a problem for the group's dynamic. As we saw in the previous chapter, the needs of an individual patient drive which practitioners are involved in care and how these practitioners interact. Each patient needs different expertise and professional activities. As a patient's needs change, members are added, while other members leave. Sometimes, this change happens frequently. Rarely is there a centralized process guiding membership in the group. Instead, practitioners are included because they fill a professional role (for instance, a social worker, a cardiologist, or an athletic trainer), and one individual may freely substitute in that role for another (see Figure 7.2). Sometimes other practitioners in the group won't even know about the addition of a new role or individual to the group of practitioners caring for a patient.

In some places, healthcare groups are more stable. Groups in clinics or rehabilitation settings often work more like typical teams that have a fixed membership and change slowly. But even with these more established groups, members need to coordinate and network their activities across multiple groups, perhaps in multiple locations, that are also trying to meet the needs of this particular patient. Group formation in healthcare is a mess, and it requires specific attention from us as frontline practitioners.

How do we adeptly navigate healthcare group formation? First, we need to try to understand the breadth of practitioners caring for an individual patient. This can include a huge number of people, dispersed across many locations; most likely, we won't be able to interact with all of these caregivers. But if we at least understand the patient's health condition and the role of other people and other groups in the care of this patient, we can network and coordinate with them successfully.

Second, we need to use our knowledge of professional roles to identify what function these practitioners fulfill in the care of the patient compared to our role. For example, if we are caring for a patient with diabetes, and our plan of care will affect the patient's diabetes, we need to identify who else—for example, the endocrinologist, the pharmacist, or the nutritionist—may have their work affected by our activities (see Figure 7.3).

Third, we need to define the group of practitioners that we should develop into a team. Across the patient's network of practitioners, some roles may be vital for close interaction, while others may not be. Some individuals who could play critical roles may have logistical barriers that limit how easily they can be integrated into a team. For example, if pharmacy expertise is important, the pharmacist down the hall may be a better team member than the pharmacist the patient sees every month at the drugstore. Or perhaps not. Developing a team takes effort, and deciding who to include involves tradeoffs. We need to be intentional about group formation and start building relationships with the right practitioners for each of our patients as we choose to have a group evolve. While typical ways of delivering care and developing groups can help us with this process, those methods may not fit with the specific needs of the patient. Pay attention to group formation; it determines how the group will evolve.

Storming

Once a group has formed, it may go through a phase known as *storming*, during which group members figure out everyone's responsibilities within the group. Sometimes, storming includes jockeying for power and testing professional boundaries. While some groups quickly pass through the storming phase, others can get stuck in it, which can hinder group performance.

In healthcare, storming is less challenging than forming, but it can be problematic. Profession-defined roles and responsibilities

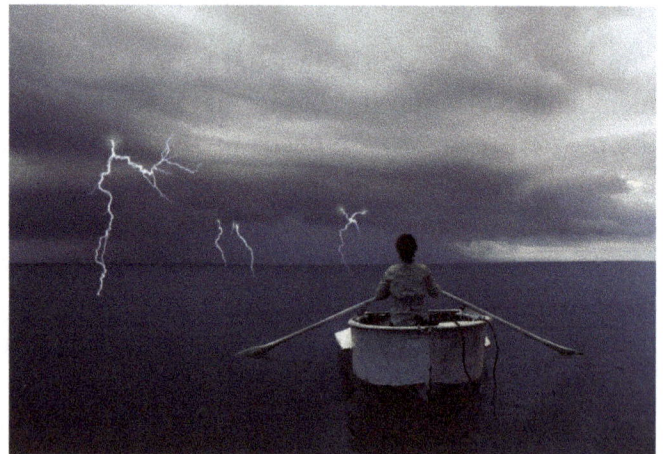
© Pavel L Photo and Video/Shutterstock.com

help to make this stage less turbulent. In addition, overarching cultural norms (see sidebar) help group members navigate the storming phase. For example, hierarchy, whether it is organizational or professional, helps group members understand how they fit together. While hierarchy can have negative effects, it smooths out the storming process. Our deeply engrained hierarchical culture in healthcare can be an advantage here.

Norms in Healthcare

Norms are the ways people typically behave in a situation. Some norms are defined by policies or rules (like professional scope of practice), while others are inherent to the culture of a location or profession. Which side of the road to drive on is a norm—the answer depends on what country you are in.

In healthcare, norms create a foundation for a shared approach to work. For example, over the past several decades, the profession of nursing has developed a strong culture of protecting and advocating for patients. Nurses often spend the most time with patients and best understand their preferences. They administer many treatments and therapies, so

Recognizing the storming phase is important for two reasons. Groups that continually engage in conflict or other struggles may be stuck in the storming phase, hampering their overall effectiveness. Identifying this problem allows the group to seek help from an external leader to clarify responsibilities and boundaries. We will discuss this more in the chapter on navigating conflict.

Additionally, groups that change too often can get stuck in a storming loop. Imagine that your group has formed and stormed and is ready to move to the next phase of its evolution. Then, a new group member is added, and the group is kicked back to the forming stage. The group must figure out how the new member fits in—the definition of storming—during which other group dynamics may also be upset. This turbulence is not the result of some interpersonal failing; rather, it is a normal result of the dynamic nature of healthcare. Whether we are part of the existing group taking on a new member or we are the new member entering a group, we have to learn how to quickly pass through the storming phase so that we can get to the work of helping the patient. Norms help us here.

Importantly, even if you work in a relatively stable group, one group member frequently changes: the patient. Your groups will constantly be reforming around each patient. Here, we storm as we identify what the patient needs, what preferences the patient has, and how those needs will be met. Our norms and roles help us here too, but we have to be ready to work differently.

Norming

Norming marks the transition between storming and performing. During norming, the group is becoming a team with a shared identity and a shared approach to work. This transition is gradual. With experience, each group member becomes better at understanding everyone else's responsibilities and preferences and how best to collaborate. Group members develop and solidify norms for interacting with each other, and these expectations lead to trust. The group may develop rituals—team huddles, particular ways of communicating, or social activities—that are part of their norms, symbolizing their shared identity (see sidebar).

Rituals

Rituals are symbolic activities that we perform as cultural traditions. We are all part of many cultures, from larger ones like our national or professional culture to smaller ones like our family's or our group's culture. Each of these cultures has activities that it does as part of its traditions. For example, your family may celebrate certain holidays with traditional activities (like regretfully eating Aunt Tillie's impenetrable Christmas fruitcake). These rituals both represent the culture and reinforce it.

Groups within workplaces have rituals too. Some groups celebrate birthdays or have going-away parties for people who are leaving. In my office, we meet once a month to talk about everyone's projects. People generally sit in the same seats, and we always go around the table clockwise. Discussion of work is mixed with humor and banter. While this process serves a function, it is also a ritual, because it symbolizes and strengthens our open and collaborative environment.

Rituals exist in clinical settings too; there, they are shaped by factors such as professional traditions and many of the drivers of collaboration that we previously discussed. For example, think about the rounding process of a medical team. The practitioners, usually physicians, medical students, and sometimes individuals from other professions, go from room to room visiting each of the patients on their team. They first gather outside the room to discuss the patient and then go into the room to talk to and examine him or her.

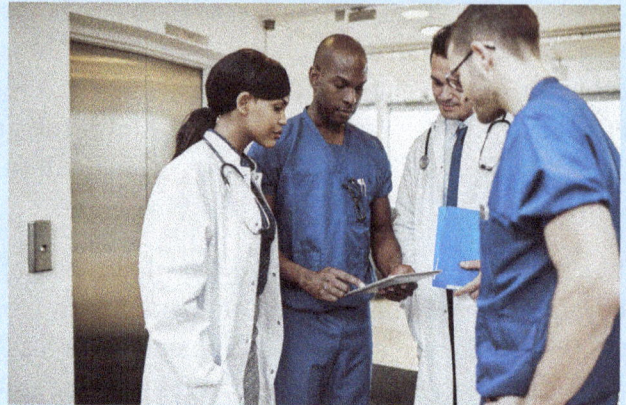

This process has a purpose—to integrate information and develop the best plan of care—but it is also a ritual with symbolic value. As a positive, it shows the team's commitment to learning from each other and having open discussions with each other. However, this ritual can also have negative implications. It can exclude nurses or other professionals, albeit unintentionally. And rounds are traditionally centered on the most senior physician's schedule rather than the patient's. For example, it's common for rounds to disrupt a patient in the midst of breakfast, bathing, or a therapy session so that the group can be efficient.

Hospitals have tried many different approaches to rounds, most of which have failed for pragmatic reasons. It's not clear what a better approach might be, but rounding is a ritual that has to balance both pragmatic constraints and the values it projects to others. Typically, the downsides of rounds have been related to external impact rather than internal functional problems.

Recognizing rituals helps identify the underlying value structure of a group and how those activities affect people—colleagues and patients—who are part of or interact with that group. Rituals both represent and reinforce culture. That's important: changing or adding rituals can be a powerful tool for altering a culture.

Norming doesn't only happen at the group level; it also happens at the individual level and across healthcare as a whole. Before we even start training as healthcare practitioners, we are norming as individuals. We see practitioners from different health professions interact on TV and in other media. We are influenced by family members and mentors from different health-related fields. And we are patients ourselves, shaped by the behaviors of the practitioners we encounter. These experiences acculturate us into healthcare and define our norms of practice. Look at how the portrayal of healthcare has evolved on television, from the physician-centric shows of the 1960s that depicted doctors as heroes to today's broader representation of professions and the more realistic representation of the emotional challenges (and comedic moments) of trying to help people.

As we go through training, our norms are strengthened and refined as we work closely with faculty and other practitioners. These norms help us navigate new situations more smoothly with new groups of practitioners and new patients. With experience, we can recall that, in a previous similar situation, a group interacted in a certain way, and this defines the norm about how we should proceed. Norms guide us through forming and storming so we can proceed with the work of patient care.

Yet norms are also fragile. When a group moves into the norming phase, some individuals might not follow the norms embraced by the rest of the group. While breaking norms based on laws, licensure, or policies can have serious ramifications, most norms are a product of an implicit culture. If some group members don't follow the same norms, the rest of the group has a choice to make: they can adjust their norms to work around the individuals who are outliers, or the group can re-enter the storming phase to redefine its norms. Breaking norms might be a good thing—it's innovation, after all—but, when done without full engagement across the group, it can be detrimental and create conflict.

Performing

Performing is the phase in group evolution where the benefits of collaboration really accrue. The group knows how to interact based on norms, and these shared approaches to work become intuitive habits. While group members will still have differences of opinion, they know how to collaborate across these differences and integrate them into a better plan for the patient.

Groups in the performing phase can have a ripple effect. Because their group members focus less effort on internal group processes, they can have more impact outside the group. Individuals from these groups may reshape norms in the other groups they collaborate with. ("This is how we approached this before, and it seemed to work.") In addition, groups in the performing phase may shape other groups through policy, training, scholarship, or quality improvement.

A big challenge of the performing phase is maintaining the group in this phase as new patients and new practitioners join an established group. The strength of the group is its norms as the group adapts its membership (revisiting the forming phase) and traverses new areas of uncertainty in interactions (via storming). A more stable membership and a clear understanding of norms among group members supports a quick resumption of the efficiency of the performing phase. While stable membership is a challenge in healthcare, our job is to try to work toward consistency of both membership and norms so that we can perform as much like a team as possible.

The other challenge in the performing phase is reluctance to change. Being part of a well-functioning team feels good, and we may not want to rock the boat. But sometimes we need to change membership or norms to better meet the needs of our patients. In the performing phase, we must be careful not to let the approach to work get stale or to exclude practitioners who could make the group even better.

Performing in a Network

As a group moves toward performing as a team, recall that practitioners outside of the group remain involved in the care of a specific patient. While these practitioners were not brought into the group in the forming stage, they stay a part of the patient's network, and the group needs to continue to interact with them to care for the patient. The group needs to identify how important these practitioners' roles are, how they should be involved in care, and what norms govern those interactions. At some point, the broader network of practitioners will likely have responsibility for the patient's care; you want them to be positioned to succeed.

Adjourning

Adjourning, the final phase of group evolution, occurs when a performing group transitions away from its close interactions. Adjourning might happen at the group level when work is concluded around a particular area or patient, such as when a patient is discharged from a hospital. Adjourning might also happen at the individual level, such as when someone leaves a group, perhaps because that person's abilities are no longer needed or because it's the end of a shift or other period of responsibility for a patient.

Adjourning is often overlooked in groups, both inside and outside of healthcare, yet we should strive to recognize the adjourning phase. Group members need to agree on how to adjourn and account for loose ends and future work, such as making sure a patient leaving the hospital has follow-up appointments, appropriate education, and new prescriptions.

It's easy for adjourning to fail. For example, in a study of nurses and doctors caring for patients at the end of life in two intensive care units, practitioners experienced more distress around these patients' care than they did caring for patients who recovered. The practitioners with more distress also rated interprofessional collaboration and the overall quality of care worse. Even though patients' deaths were inevitable, better collaboration might have improved care and made the practitioners feel less distressed about the loss. This failure to use interprofessional collaboration to achieve closure around the loss of patients represents a missed opportunity to provide better care to patients and strengthen the ongoing relationships between group members.

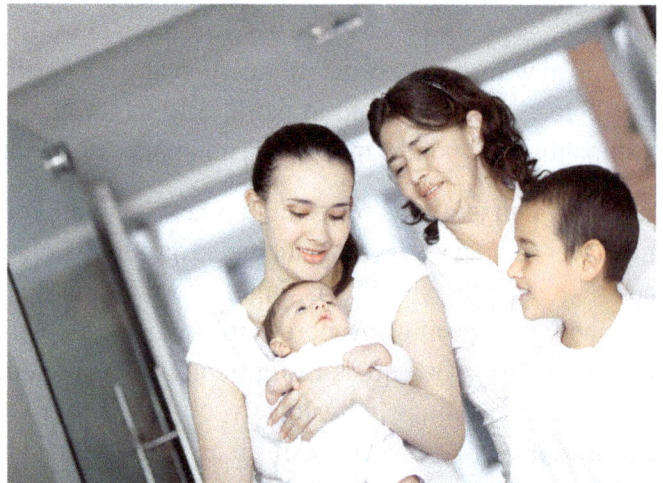

This example highlights the key point about adjourning: with the way that groups form, dissolve, and reform in healthcare, adjourning is often temporary. Recognizing an end by adjourning helps set the stage for future interactions and lets us think about how we might work together better in the future. We are likely to be working together again soon.

Application Questions

Thinking about your ideal job in healthcare, identify several diverse groups of which you might be a part. Reference the drivers of collaboration from the previous chapter if you need help thinking about different types of groups.

> Which of these groups, if any, have the potential to form into teams, and which groups will likely only interact as networks? Why might one of these groups begin to become more closely connected and move through the stage of group evolution? How might the members of this group be selected?

> What are some issues around unclear roles and responsibilities that might lead to storming?

> What are some norms that might shape how this group interacts? If you can, describe a ritual that reinforces some of these norms?

Why might this group adjourn?

Final Reflection Questions

Imagine that you are a longstanding member of a group. Most of the other members have been with the group for a while too. Organizational leaders have recently added a new member to the team, and, since the addition of this new member, your group has spent a lot of time reviewing and discussing the way the group functions. The new member has brought a number of new ideas to the group, and many of the old members are hesitant to change the way the group functions.

How you would describe this group's stage of evolution?

What are the benefits of the new member's ideas? How do they fit in with our concept of group evolution?

What are the benefits of the hesitancy of the old members? How do their perspectives fit in with our concept of group evolution?

How might you resolve this situation?

We discussed that norms are often based on how people behave rather than specific rules or policies. What are some approaches to supporting positive norms? What approaches might be used to change problematic norms and alter the overall culture of a setting?

Further Reading

Bruce Tuckman originally described his stages of group development in the publication "Developmental Sequence in Small Groups" in the *Psychological Bulletin* in 1965. Subsequently, the model has been refined, including adding the adjourning stage, which did not appear in the original publication. However, the original publication is a good place to start if you want to read more about Tuckman's framework.

Moral distress is the term used to describe the emotions that come from the conflict between what a person believes is right and what is being done. In healthcare, moral distress has been best described within the ethical quandaries of ICU care, particularly when care seems to be futile (i.e., not likely to benefit a patient with a poor prognosis or functional status). Ann Hamric and Leslie Blackhall's publication "Nurse-Physician Perspectives on the Care of Dying Patients in Intensive Care Units: Collaboration, Moral Distress, and Ethical Climate" in *Critical Care Medicine*, 2007, is a good place to begin to learn more about moral distress and how it relates to interprofessional collaboration.

CHAPTER 8

Group Process and Coordination

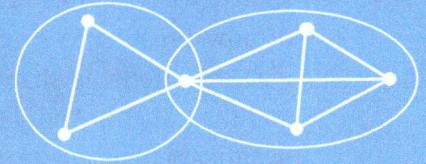

Now that we've talked about the different types of groups and about how groups evolve, let's look at how groups should ideally collaborate. When group members collaborate, they are most commonly planning individual activities. In this chapter, we will look at a framework that describes how group members conduct the shared work of planning and then complete the independent work of doing the planned individual activities. This framework will provide the final piece of the foundation for understanding groups as we head into the next section of the book on techniques for interacting in various collaborative situations. By the end of this chapter, you should be able to:

▸ compare and contrast the planning and action phases of group work;
▸ discuss the importance of reviewing past performance of group work;
▸ describe the role of contingency plans in shaping group work; and
▸ relate the planning and action phases to the three different types of collaboration: teamwork, coordination, and networking.

Initial Reflection Questions

Think about a time when you were part of a group working toward a shared goal. This could have been with a team or some other, looser form of collaboration.

What activities were performed collectively, meaning the group all did them together?

What activities were performed individually, meaning group members did them alone?

How did the collective activities influence the individual activities? Was there some method by which collective activities shaped what the individuals did as part of their individual activities?

How did the individual activities shape the collective activities? Was there feedback from the individual activities to the overall group?

Group Process and Coordination

Across the spectrum of collaboration—networking, coordination, and teamwork—both individual activities and shared work are important. Healthcare practitioners need a common understanding of what a patient needs and how those needs will be met. While teamwork by definition involves shared work, networking and coordination also require at least a shared model of how practitioners' individual activities fit together to help each patient. How well this model is shared across practitioners impacts the outcomes of the group and the patient. And, because networking and coordination are more common in healthcare than true teamwork, we need an overarching model to guide our shared work, regardless of the type of collaboration.

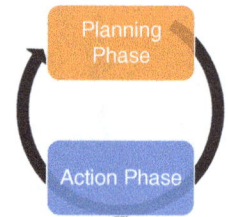

Figure 8.1 The Two Phases of the Group Process Model. Source: Alan Dow.

Let's examine the model in Figure 8.1. This model was originally called the "Team Process Model," but I will use the term *group* so that we don't muddy the waters with the term *team*. In the model, group process consists of two alternating phases: the planning phase and the action phase. Let's explore each phase and then relate this model to the different types of collaboration.

The Planning Phase

The group works collectively in the planning phase. The activities of this phase might be thought of as teamwork though that episode may be brief. In the planning phase, the group decides what individual activities will occur in the next action phase, but the group has several key tasks to perform in the planning phase in order to make those decisions.

Planning Phase Activities:

- Review past performance
- Identify external considerations
- Set goals for action phase
- Define responsibilities of group members
- Plan follow-up and contingencies

First, the group needs to review its past performance. In healthcare, the status of the patient is the most central information. Each group member brings a profession-specific assessment of the patient's status and needs during the upcoming action phase. The group may pull from past experience either in caring for this patient or in working with each other and other patients in this setting.

In addition, the group should think about how it is performing as a group. This is the time to make suggestions about how to improve the group's overall function. Anyone in the group may have a great idea to improve the group's work, and the planning phase provides a venue to bring up these ideas and decide whether and how to work differently. This is an essential aspect of the most successful groups: they consciously think about how to work better. We often skip this aspect of group work in healthcare.

During the planning phase, the group should also identify considerations external to the group that might affect the group's work. Some considerations might be institutional initiatives. For example, most hospitals have efforts to increase the number of patients discharged before noon. The planning phase provides a venue for the group to integrate that institutional priority into its work. Another consideration might be environmental constraints. A hospital might have a shortage of a certain medication. That information might be brought to the planning phase of a group, say by a pharmacist, who might describe the shortage and recommend some alternatives. The planning phase is the time to integrate this essential external information into the group's work.

Once the group has considered the patient's status, the group's prior performance, and any external considerations, the next activities of the planning phase are to set goals and define the activities for each group member in the subsequent action phase. Integrating all the information the group has received from various sources, group members should define what the group hopes to accomplish and who will do which activities—the professional responsibilities—in the next action phase. Decisions about who has responsibility for each activity should integrate not only professional scope of practice but also each member's workload, ability, and interest. For the group to perform optimally, group members need to ensure that work is shared fairly and appopriately. The process of setting goals and designating responsibilities can be challenging; we will spend several chapters discussing shared decision-making (chapter 9) and conflict navigation (chapter 11). However, our norms can help us navigate this process smoothly and efficiently.

As a last step before re-entering the action phase, the group should decide on plans for follow-up and contingencies. Many, but not all, groups have standard times (a norm) for the next group meeting: for example, daily huddles and weekly conferences. Defining when and where the next planning phase will occur is essential for keeping the group stable and for continuing to collaborate effectively. The group should also anticipate challenges that might arise during the action phase and develop contigency plans. That way, should a challenge arise, group members are already be prepared to pivot from their individual responsibilities to solve the problem. Sometimes, responding to a challenge requires reconvening some or all of the group members in a mini-planning phase; that's a reasonable contigency plan if input from several group members is needed. What's important is to identify potential issues and decide ahead of time how best to work through these challenges so that the patient's overall care is not derailed and the planned work of the action phase continues.

With new patients or new group members, expect the planning process to take longer. The group needs to traverse storming and norming (see chapter 7) as they learn how to work together efficiently in the planning phase. And we need a good plan before proceeding.

The Action Phase

In the action phase, members of the group perform their typical professional activities as defined by the planning phase. These activities are what we usually think of as the work of a healthcare practitioner: evaluating a patient, administering treatment, providing patient education, and so on. Usually, these activities are done individually, although sometimes group members can work together in subgroups.

Action Phase Activities:

- Individual professional activities
- Monitoring of progress
- Adapting to changing conditions
- Identifying concerns for future planning phases

But other activities should also occur in the action phase. Group members should monitor the progress of their own work and of the other group members they interact with. If someone's progress is delayed or ahead of schedule, group members might need to alter what they are doing or change how they are interacting. For example, an inpatient nurse may need to schedule medication administration around a therapy visit. Group members need to adapt their professional activities to the changing conditions of work, which demands an awareness of those conditions.

Group members should also think about how the group is functioning overall. If the group seems to be falling short in some way, group members should notice and bring this concern to the group.

While some changes can be made quickly and easily, other changes require discussion with the broader group because they influence the work of many people and may have unintended consequences. These observations are provided as feedback to the group, which brings us back to the planning phase.

Examples of the Group Process Model

Let's examine the group process model in action in several settings to see how it can help us collaborate better.

Group Process in a Subacute Nursing Facility

Think about a patient in a subacute nursing facility (SNF). A typical SNF patient is trying to recover after a serious medical event such as a car crash, stroke, or surgery. These patients stay in the SNF for an average of three weeks to do therapy that will increase their functional status. The goal is for them to go home and live as independently as possible.

The group of practitioners caring for a typical SNF patient include a physical therapist, an occupational therapist, a speech therapist, a bachelor's-prepared nursing leader, several nursing aides, and a nursing home administrator. This group might meet twice a week to review all of the patients on the unit. This meeting serves as their planning phase.

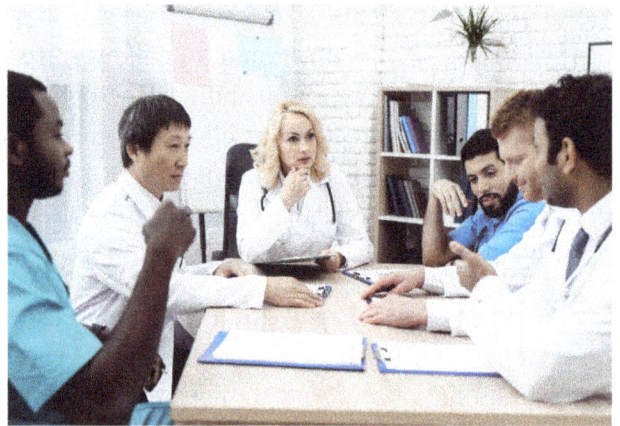

© VGstockstudio/Shutterstock.com

The nursing leader and nursing home administrator might start the meeting by commenting on external considerations like staffing concerns or facilities issues. Then, one group member might present an assessment and plan for the first patient. Other group members add additional input as needed on that patient. For new patients, this process may take longer than it does for older patients, but with older patients, the group also discusses whether it met the goals set at the last meeting. The group then defines new goals for the patient to achieve between this meeting and the next one, and each member identifies how he or she will help the patient meet those goals. While a therapist might work on initially teaching a patient an exercise, the nursing aides may assume the key responsibility of reinforcing that teaching and monitoring progress. Finally, the group discusses any potential challenges between this meeting and the next and makes contigency plans for those challenges. Having completed planing on this patient, the group members then discuss the next patient. After all the patients have been reviewed, the group enters the action phase, ready to meet the group's new goals for each patient.

Think about where this process can go wrong. It might be that the meeting never happens because the planning phase is not recognized as important. Or some activities of the planning phase could be missed: a leader could fail to raise the appropriate external considerations, the group could falter at devising shared goals or a shared approach to achieving these goals, or the group could not identify potential challenges and contingency plans. In any of these cases, the group is not set up to be completely successful.

Group Process in an Intensive Care Unit

As another example, consider a group in the intensive care unit (ICU). The physicians and pharmacists in the group might round together on each patient every day. As this group arrives outside each patient's room, the nurse for that patient joins the group.

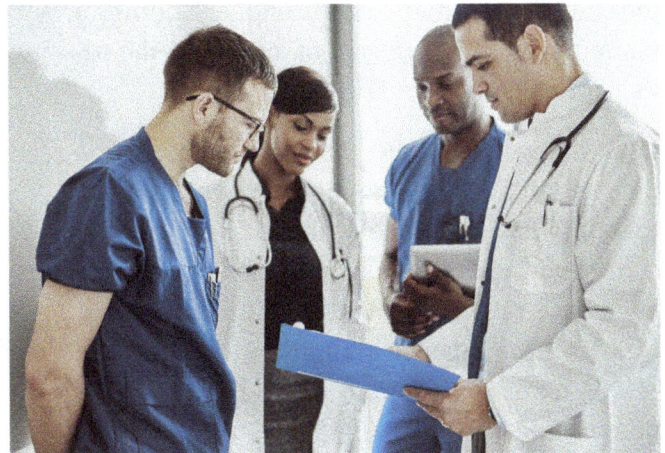

© Flamingo Images/Shutterstock.com

Together, they conduct a daily planning phase where they review the patient's progress from each of their perspectives, discuss the goals for the upcoming day, and identify everyone's responsibilities for that day. Group members can voice any external constraints or possible areas of concern that might require contingency planning. The group members can then proceed into the action phase for that patient with each member recognizing that another planning phase may be necessary, such as if the patient's conditions worsens.

In contrast to a SNF, membership in the group changes between patients. Some of the planning phase activities must occur in a different forum. Instead of discussing every external consideration or revising the group's process during rounds, the unit might have monthly meetings to talk about group performance across the unit and review how they might improve the process of the rounding across the entire unit. If these monthly meeting are not held and prioritized, the groups will not improve. Here, the group process model helps us think about how collaboration should look and what elements should be integrated to ensure optimal collaboration.

Group Process for Integrating a Psychologist in Primary Care

Now think about the integration of a new psychologist into an established primary care practice. This is an example of group process driving change by creating new norms. The psychologist and the primary care practitioners (PCPs) decide to meet weekly to talk about how they can best collaborate. At each meeting (the planning phase), the psychologist and the PCPs review patients that they share or that they could possibly share in the future. While the clinical work around the patients is important, more essential at this point is developing a shared approach to work.

Each group member identifies the challenges and constraints surrounding their shared care—issues such as handing off patients, communicating around plans of care, and maintaining professional boundaries. They then plan the activities in the action phase to test approaches to collaboration and solve challenges that might arise through contigency plans. The group is developing norms for a better group process that will lead to better patient care. The group process model drives how they are learning to work together and helps define everyone's responsibilities in each phase of the model.

Group Process for Home-Based Care

Finally, think about a physical therapist visiting patients in their homes. The therapist is in the action phase, executing plans devised by an interprofessional group of practitioners during a planning phase with a goal of increasing the patients' functional status.

Let's imagine that the therapist encounters a patient who has a new medical concern. The therapist has to decide which of a number of contigency plans to pursue: offering reassurance, referring the patient to primary care, or calling an ambulance. While the therapist had been working in a network as part of the action phase, he or she can move into a planning phase with closer collaboration just by picking up the phone. And that planning phase may lead to a number of possible action phases with a variety of collaborators.

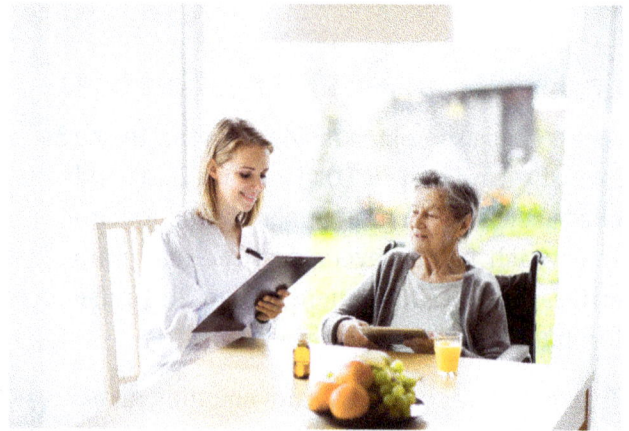

© Halfpoint/Shutterstock.com

While the action phase often involves networking or coordination, the planning phase usually requires closer collaboration. Group members in the action phase work more independently with little or no interaction. But they are tethered together by a shared approach to work, including the knowledge that they may reconvene as a team in a future planning phase.

Group Process and Group Failure

These different examples demonstrate that the group process framework can be molded to fit across many contexts. While the phases and the activities within them are consistent, the way that this idea is applied to a specific group in a certain context varies. This framework gives you a way to categorize the activities of collaboration and identify what may be lacking as you strive to collaborate more effectively.

While groups can fail because of conflict in the planning phase or incompetence in the action phase, interprofessional collaboration more commonly fails because the structure for group process is lacking. Frequently, the planning phase is poorly structured or nonexistent. Group members may not recognize the planning phase as essential for other group members to perform at their best. Leadership and advocacy are essential here to develop a functional structure for the group to succeed (see sidebar). The planning phase takes an investment of time, but that investment pays dividends in terms of outcomes and efficiency. The planning phase develops accountability and group identity, which can then spur the group's future evolution toward becoming a team. Group process is not always easy or even possible, but this framework is a blueprint for a group's success.

Leadership and the Group

Note the role of leadership in the various activities of the group process model. While certain individuals may be formally recognized as leaders because of professional or organizational status in the hierarchy, everyone can be a leader in this model. Every group member can identify concerns, suggest ideas for improving team performance, and communicate key information from external sources. This has important implications for how we think about leadership.

Leadership has often been considered an individual characteristic, but more and more it is being recognized as a group characteristic. A group that has a vibrant exchange of ideas and a collaborative approach to problem solving has a high leadership capacity. On the other hand, a group with low leadership capacity might have group members who are not invested or who don't effectively collaborate to solve problems or resolve conflicts.

If leadership is a group characteristic, how can you as an individual enhance the group's leadership capacity? Even if you don't have a formal leadership role, recognize your role as a leader. The group needs your thoughtful opinions and expertise and, as you bring these to the group, you will increasingly be acknowledged as a leader. And, when you do have a formal leadership role, use that authority to empower others and include their perspectives. The most effective leaders often set aside their opinions to help the group move forward. They know having stronger leadership distributed across the team is more important for the group in the long term. If we're only as strong as our weakest link, we need to help all our colleagues become a strong link.

Application Questions

Thinking about your current or desired work setting, describe the group process that will occur. Specifically:

When and where does the planning phase take place? Is it well defined or is it lacking in structure?

Does the group review its past performance? How does the group work to improve future performance?

How are external considerations integrated into the group's decision-making process? Can you identify any examples?

How does the group decide on plans and assign responsibilities for the next action phase?

Can you describe examples of contingency plans within this group?

Based on your example above, how might your groups work better? What gaps have you identified in group process, and what approaches might fill these gaps? What are the downsides of your suggested approaches?

Final Reflection Questions

When I described the ICU as having both rounding and monthly meetings to discuss overall unit performance, it was an example of a small group process embedded in a larger group process. Similarly, the physical therapist visiting a patient at home may belong to just one of many cycles of group process surrounding that patient. What different levels or cycles of group process might be embedded in your current or future work environment? How does the work at each different level of group process interact with other work to shape the overall care of the patient? Think about the different drivers of collaboration discussed in chapter 6.

I described leadership as a group characteristic. Can you identify a group you were involved in that had high group leadership? What about one that had low group leadership? What factors contributed to the difference in group leadership between these groups?

Further Reading

The framework for group process at the center of this chapter was originally described in the article "A Temporally Based Framework and Taxonomy of Team Process," by Michelle Marks, John Mathieu, and Stephen Zaccaro, published in *The Academy of Management Review* in 2001.

My colleagues and I applied this framework to healthcare in a 2013 article in *Academic Medicine*, "Applying Organizational Science to Health Care: A Framework for Collaborative Practice."

If you want to read more about leadership as a team characteristic, start with "Leadership in Teams: A Functional Approach to Understanding Leadership Structures and Processes," by Frederick Morgeson, Scott DeRue, and Elizabeth Karam, published in *The Journal of Management* in 2010.

SECTION 4

The Process of Interprofessional Practice

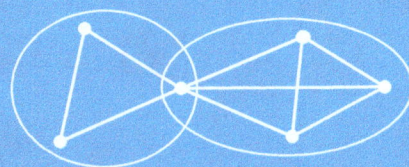

CHAPTER 9

Group Decision-Making

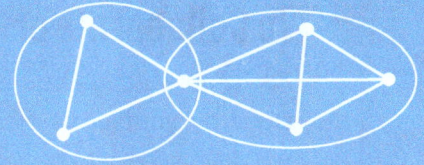

We've now looked at the basic building blocks of healthcare collaboration, including the roles and responsibilities of individuals from different professions, some structures for how these individuals interact, and some frameworks for how these groups evolve and collaborate. The rest of the book will focus on specific elements of communication and provide some guidance for how to use these skills in the moment to collaborate more effectively.

The focus of this chapter is the different ways groups make decisions. As we noted in previous chapters, healthcare practitioners work in dynamic groups with changing memberships and patterns of interaction. Yet an essential piece of collaboration is that these groups make collective decisions to help their patients. This is the key output of the planning phase of group process. Understanding the different ways in which groups make decisions and how to make better decisions as a group will help you engage more effectively in the decision-making process and make better decisions for your patients. By the end of this chapter, you will be able to:

▸ outline an approach for consensus decision-making,
▸ understand the benefits and challenges of dissenting opinions in group decision-making, and
▸ compare and contrast the effects of different types of decision-making in healthcare.

Initial Reflection Questions

Imagine that you are going out to dinner with a group of friends or family members. How do you decide where to go? Under what circumstances might one person unilaterally pick a restaurant? What are the advantages and disadvantages of this approach?

What are the circumstances under which multiple people might be involved in picking a restaurant? What are the advantages and disadvantages of this approach?

Why might someone not voice an opinion at all? What are the advantages and disadvantages of someone staying quiet?

To Collaborate or Not to Collaborate

As important as groups can be, making decisions by yourself is essential in healthcare. As we discussed when we talked about the types of work, you've had years of training to become a capable healthcare practitioner. You are an expert, and your patients are counting on your expertise to help them. Most decisions at work are ones that you will make by yourself.

Individual decision-making has its benefits. It's efficient and usually not strenuous. Your patients and colleagues expect that you are working competently as an individual within your scope of practice. In some ways, that's the easy part of healthcare.

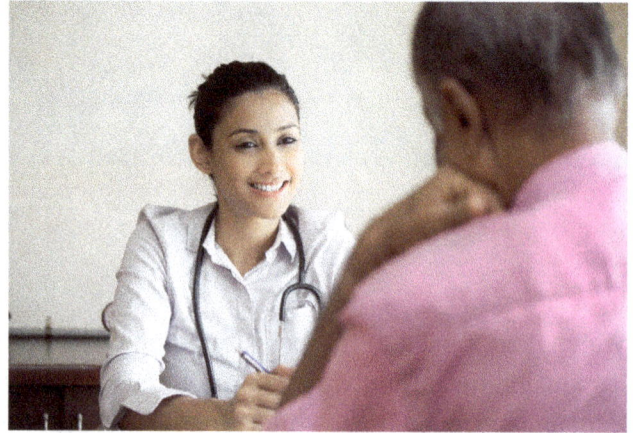

© AshTproductions/Shutterstock.com

Individual decision-making has downsides though. Individual decisions are not made in isolation. Because we work in groups, our decisions interact with the decisions of other practitioners and affect the work of other practitioners. Sometimes these complex interactions can turn a correct individual decision into the wrong overall decision (see sidebar).

Garbage In, Garbage Out

Within the complex environment of healthcare, sometimes we fail to recognize the impact of our individual actions on downstream patient care. Other times, we can erroneously act on incorrect information to propagate a mistake. Let me give you an example.

At my hospital, we identified the importance of accurate patient weights for professional activities like determining medication doses. The challenge was that patients were being weighed on clinical units, while medication doses were being confirmed in the pharmacy, away from the patient on the clinical units (an example of networking). To ensure that we had accurate weights, we developed a policy requiring that a practitioner ordering a medication must also enter that patient's weight. This policy included a rule in the electronic health record that enforced the policy. While this seemed like a good solution, let's look at what happened.

In the emergency department, among other places, many patients were too ill or uncomfortable to be weighed. Other patients might be unconscious or agitated. Practitioners were left with a choice. Some entered an estimated weight that was basically just a guess. While these weights were marked as estimates, they seemed reasonable, and other practitioners, like the pharmacists, would presume that they were correct. Unfortunately, these errors in weight entry led to errors in medication dosing that could have harmed patients.

Other practitioners, rather than guessing at a weight, entered an outlandish number, usually 1 kilogram, as an indicator to everyone that the weight was made up. Now, no one presumed that the number was right, but the erroneous weight didn't solve the original networking problem of needing a weight for medication dosing. This is an example of a *workaround* where a well-intentioned solution is cumbersome so people on the frontline 'work around' the solution to complete their other responsibilities.

We continue to try to solve this problem of having accurate patient weights in the electronic health record. With a number of other interventions, we've gotten much better, but the fundamental problem remains that the individual professional activity of weighing a patient has broad and surprising ramifications across our network.

Individual decision-making might also be less safe. All of us make mistakes—human error is, after all, human. Fortunately, whether we are working closely within a team or more dispersed in a network, our colleagues and other safeguards often catch errors before they can harm a patient. But we have an added layer of protection when we are collaborating closely. A common example is the requirement for double-checking by two nurses before the administration of a high-risk medication. One way to make fewer individual errors is to recognize when the individual decision-making is more difficult. When individual decision-making becomes strenuous, that's a signal you might need help.

However, the biggest downside to individual decision-making is that you, the individual, lose out on the expertise of the rest of the group. The special knowledge, abilities, and understanding of the patient that your colleagues bring to the group are the most important benefits of collaborative decision-making. For example, imagine I've prescribed a certain medication to a patient. The medication is the right drug at the right dose for the right problem. I think I've nailed it. But then I get a call from a pharmacist in the community. The medication that I prescribed is not covered by this patient's insurance. By failing to consider the formulary of the patient's insurance, I've made an error that could end up costing the patient. Fortunately, the pharmacist had access to this information, identified the potential problem, and called me so that we could dispense a similar, cheaper medication from the formulary. Initially, I made the medication decision as an individual, but the pharmacist engaged with me in group decision-making to add his or her expertise. This took a little bit of time for both of us, but it resulted in better patient care because we combined our expertise.

Individual decision-making is critical to healthcare. It is how you will work most of the time, guided by your scope of practice. It is efficient and essential to the care of patients. But it's not perfect, and you should understand when and how to enter into group decision-making to best meet your patients' needs. Collaboration takes time and effort, and you and your colleagues are busy. Collaboration can be especially challenging when you do not have a clearly defined planning phase and an opportunity to discuss issues together. Often, we have to be intentional about deciding to collaborate.

Group Decision-Making

In healthcare, we enter into group decision-making in several ways. We may have formal planning phases that support group decision-making. Other times, group decision-making may flow spontaneously from the way we work. Finally, the most challenging way to enter into group decision-making is when we have to urgently form an unexpected group to implement a better plan for a patient in crisis. Let's take a closer look at examples of these ways of engaging in group decision-making.

Planning phase processes such as meetings or huddles exist to support group decision-making because we know groups make better decisions than individuals on questions that don't have straightforward answers. These meetings usually focus on complex, recurring questions, such as:

- How can we help this patient after he or she leaves the hospital?
- How should we support this child with complex health needs so he or she can thrive in school?
- Have we ensured that this patient's operations will go as smoothly as possible?

These forums are important venues for group decision-making because they support the sharing of diverse opinions and collaborating on the next steps in care. They are the ideal.

Alternatively, we may engage in group decision-making in healthcare when our professional activities rely on each other (as described in chapter 3). Consider an occupational therapist and a speech therapist working individually with a patient who had a stroke to improve his ability to eat. The occupational therapist might focus on the patient's ability to get food from his plate to his mouth, while the speech therapist focuses on his ability to swallow that food. Each therapist needs to consider the other's opinion on how the patient can best navigate these distinct activities, such as opinions on the consistency of the food and the devices he can use to help with eating. The practitioners should have a conversation with each other to come up with joint recommendations. This type of interaction could be considered a mini-planning phase or collaborative work in the action phase. It's probably the most common form of group decision-making in healthcare.

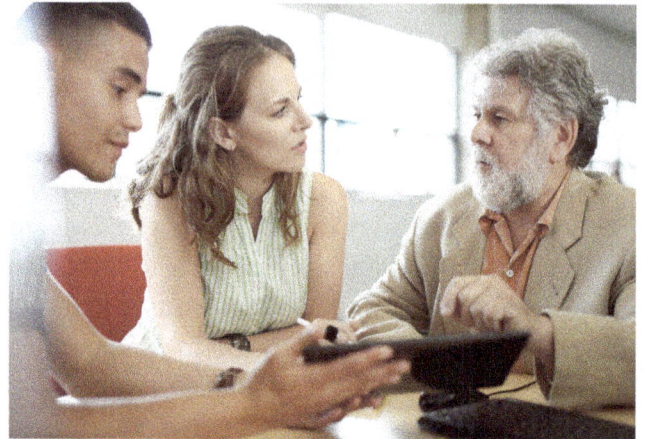

On the other hand, the most acute way that we engage in group decision-making is when one health practitioner unexpectedly brings together one or more colleagues to make a group decision. Although this is a common pathway to group decision-making, it's not necessarily easy. When this happens, people are pulled away from their other work responsibilities, and there can be some interpersonal challenges. In the example above, the pharmacist noted that I had made an error around the formulary on the patient's insurance and saw an opportunity to improve patient care. While the pharmacist did the right thing, that collaborative activity takes effort and can be challenging: the pharmacist did not know how I would react to a suggestion about a prescription. All of us want to provide the best care for our patients, but we don't always receive feedback well (see Chapter 12). Great collaboration sometimes requires us to pull colleagues into group decision-making unexpectedly, and that may be difficult.

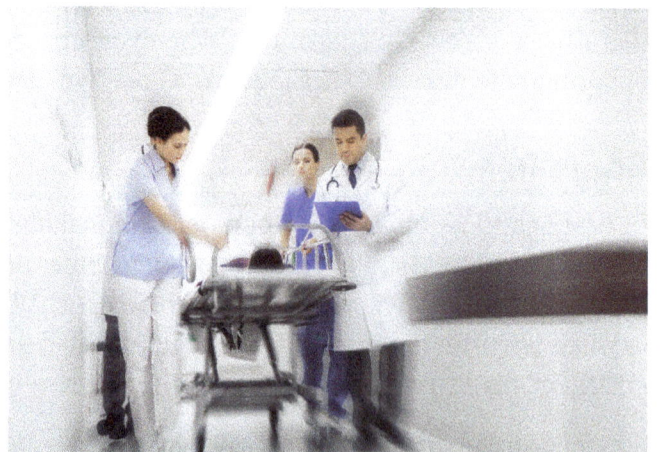

You need more than individual decision-making to help patients. Regular planning phases and natural collaboration support group decision-making. Collaboration that is more atypical and unplanned has a greater potential for difficult interpersonal dynamics. Regardless of the type, all group decision-making always takes effort. Let's look at an approach to group decision-making that can help you make the most of this effort and navigate the more challenging aspects of this process of making group decisions.

Consensus Decision-Making

Consensus decision-making is a model for group decision-making that involves several steps (see Figure 9.1). While this model may seem overly complex for relatively straightforward group decision-making, its principles can be useful even in making simple decisions. Let's spend a moment examining each step and thinking about how this model can apply to all sorts of group decisions.

Form Your Group – The first step in consensus decision-making is deciding who should be in the group. You are familiar with this concept from our discussion of group evolution in Chapter 7. Remember that both the relationship with the patient and the scopes of practice of different practitioners should help define who should be in the group. The patient or a family member is often essential here but sometimes overlooked.

Decide whether and how external leaders should help with forming the group; if you may need the help of external leaders later, don't forget to engage them early. Some people may have a role advising the group but don't necessarily need to be part of the final decision. The key element of this step is thinking about who is important for shaping and making the decision so you don't have to revisit this step later. You can always add people as needed, but for complex, significant decisions, asking your colleagues at the outset who else should be involved can be a good idea so you don't have to return to the forming (and storming) phase.

Define the Issue and Express Perspectives – Defining the issue and expressing perspectives about it may be done concurrently. Each group member might not define the issue in a similar way. Some may not have a full understanding of the issue. By letting group members express their perspectives, the group develops a common understanding of the issue and can focus its attention on the critical differences that are the areas where decision-making is needed.

While some group members can be impatient to make a decision, spending time on this task saves time later in the decision-making process. It is important to develop guiding norms, like those created in a formal planning phase, to encourage efficiency and respect. The urgency of making a decision is

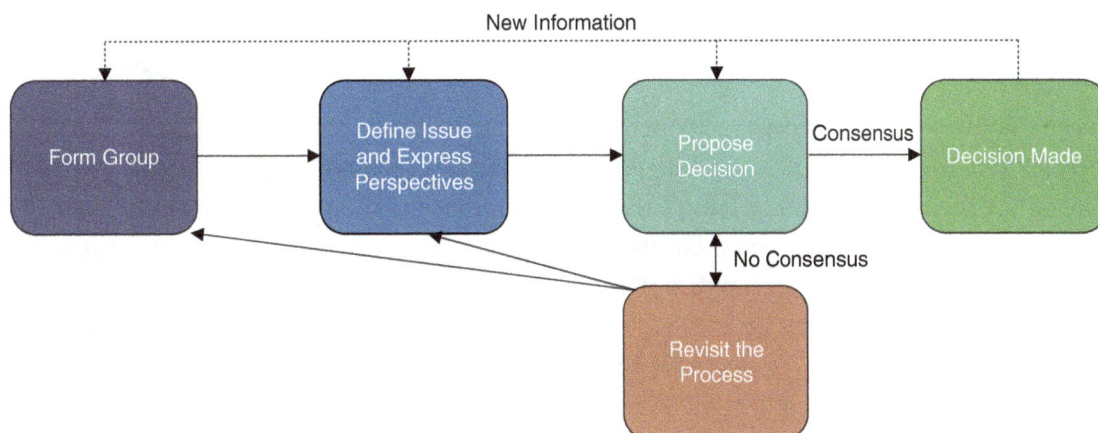

Figure 9.1 A Framework for Consensus Decision-Making. Source: Alan Dow.

one of the important perspectives here, but needlessly rushing the process and failing to agree on the issue can make the decision process take much longer and create needless conflict.

Leadership is critical. Whoever convened the group will be seen as a leader, as will group members who have more experience or who are higher in the traditional professional hierarchy. However, anyone can demonstrate leadership by encouraging others, especially the less empowered, to express their perspectives while still moving the decision-making process forward. One useful approach to guide a discussion is agenda-setting (sidebar).

Propose Decision – Once the issue has been defined and group members have contributed what they think is necessary to the discussion, it's time to make a decision. Decisions are unlikely to be straightforward, or you wouldn't need to participate in this complicated process. Often, various options have competing benefits and downsides: for example, you may be stuck selecting the best of several bad options. If you are leading the group and proposing a path forward, start by doing two things:

1. **Articulate where there appears to be clear agreement on how to move forward.** Make sure that everyone agrees on these points. This approach helps to shrink the scope of discussion to the most challenging issues.

2. **Propose a course of action for the less certain areas without expecting that your proposal is the best approach.** Describe your rationale and incorporate the advantages and disadvantages of that choice in the context of other possible choices. Having a proposed course of action helps the group focus its discussion. For sure, the group will change and improve on your proposed course of action—that's the point of having a group decision in the first place—and you need to be willing to listen to everyone's feedback and adjust your proposal.

> **Agenda-Setting**
>
> Agenda-setting is a useful technique for guiding a discussion with other people, whether it be an interprofessional meeting or a visit with a patient. Agenda-setting is the first task in a discussion. It entails defining what everyone wants to talk about and how much time is going to be spent on each topic. Sometimes there isn't time to cover all issues. If so, each person should at least have his or her most pressing issue discussed.
>
> By having a road map for the discussion, each person knows how quickly and at what depth to proceed through each part of the discussion. In addition, agenda-setting support equity and respect by giving everyone a chance to have his or her most important issue addressed. Not only is the approach useful in interprofessional collaboration, it is essential during short-duration clinical visits where the goal is to provide patient-centered care while also addressing the clinical priorities of each patient.

Throughout the approach, leaders should ensure that everyone feels heard. At this point, the group can either have consensus or no consensus. Bear in mind that consensus is not equivalent to contentment. Compromise generally means that everyone is equally unhappy about a decision.

No Consensus: Revisit the Process – Not achieving consensus raises several questions. Each of these questions centers on the issue of what the person (or persons) who has prevented consensus wants. This concept of the intention underlying the position of dissent is one that we will discuss in depth during the later chapters of this book. For example, the person preventing consensus might feel that the proposed solution is not ideal and that the group needs more information or more discussion and should return to an earlier step in the decision-making process. Counterbalancing the notion of revisiting the process to reach consensus is the urgency of making a decision. It is also possible that this person wants to voice an objection to the proposed decision but can offer no better course of action; this person may be willing to see the decision carried out as long as it's clear that he or she is uncomfortable with it. Often, a side conversation with the dissenter can define the issue. Questions to consider include these:

1. **Does the group need to integrate additional perspectives or expertise?** Perhaps the dissenter is right that the group needs some additional input. The dissenter may have an unheard perspective or may think someone else from outside the group needs to provide input. The group may be engaged in *groupthink*, which is reaching consensus because of the desire to agree. New perspectives are the antidote to groupthink (see sidebar).

2. **Does everyone feel heard?** Sometimes individuals have not had a chance to voice their concerns or to offer a different course of action. As long as they feel understood and have registered their discomfort, they may be willing to allow a group's decision-making process to move forward.

3. **How urgent is this decision?** Sometimes individuals, especially patients, just need time to consider a decision. That's OK, but not achieving consensus and thus not making a decision is a type of decision: the decision not to decide (yet). This decision ensures the status quo, which might be a bad decision, particularly for the patient. Restating the urgency to make a decision as described in Step 2 can sometimes push the group toward consensus.

Dissent: The Antidote to Groupthink

Dissenting opinions are essential for optimal group decision-making. If the diversity of perspectives and expertise are the strengths of a group, the biggest danger with group decision-making is groupthink. Groupthink is when a group makes poor decisions because of a failure to incorporate all the wisdom and diverse perspectives of the group. Groupthink can occur for two reasons:

1. Group members fail to bring up objections or alternatives because they do not want to put effort into making the best group decision.
2. Group members fail to express different opinions because they feel uncomfortable expressing these opinions.

Either reason can be looked at as a failure of leadership.

Leaders should ensure that group members are actively engaged in decision-making. Group members should understand the importance of the decision-making process and each person's role in contributing to decisions. After all, forming the group takes effort and that effort shouldn't be wasted on disengaged decision-making. In addition, leaders should ensure that everyone feels comfortable expressing their opinions, a concept known as *psychological safety*. Leaders can support psychological safety and encourage less empowered group members through techniques such as asking specifically for their input, validating their contributions, and managing interactions with group members who may seek to disempower others. The important point is to make sure that dissenting opinions are heard so that the group can consider these perspectives and integrate them into the final group decisions.

Not Deciding

One way that group decision-making fails is by not reaching a decision at all. Faced with a tough situation, a group may get stuck not having consensus. But recognize this: not making a decision is making a decision for the status quo. Continuing on the same course might be the right decision: perhaps changing course is not urgent, or more time is needed to understand the issue. But not deciding needs to be recognized as a decision that may have consequences.

When the decision is to not decide, the group should consider these questions: When will the decision be revisited? What information might help us decide differently? What changes would increase the urgency of making a different decision? Outlining these parameters will help the group work more effectively as it continues to consider other courses of action.

If a group is stuck, you may need the help of external leaders. As we will see when we talk about conflict in chapter 11, sometimes irresolvable conflict needs help from beyond the immediate group. If a decision has to be made and your group won't make one, it's time to get help.

A Decision—Finally?

The group has made a decision. Now what? Functionally, the group must transition into the action phase, but that's not the only aspect of the group to pay attention to. Consensus decision-making can be hard—remember, everyone might leave feeling equally unhappy. Paying attention to the group's dynamics and nurturing morale is important. You may have just traversed a hard period of storming and developed some new norms. How can you use those norms to help the group make better decisions in the future? This question can be worth a wrap-up discussion with the group.

In addition, remember that decisions need not be final. Healthcare is dynamic and, as circumstances change, a decision might also need to be changed. Consider contingency plans such as parameters that might be defined to reconvene the group to revisit a decision. The goal is to make the best decisions and to do so efficiently, even as the patient's needs continue to evolve.

Other Types of Group Decision-Making

Groups make decisions in many other ways. Think about politics. We vote, and the majority rules. Sometimes a supermajority (like 60 percent) is needed for certain legislative actions. And, sometimes, committed dissenters can stop a decision from being made. While most of these approaches don't have much relevance for direct healthcare delivery, they are important to recognize and may have value in certain leadership contexts.

One other type of group decision-making that does happen in healthcare is decision-making by a privileged few. This is an alternative to consensus decision-making and represents a failure of collaboration. A common example occurs when physicians make decisions without involving other healthcare practitioners. In later chapters, we will look at hierarchy and advocacy and how to handle a situation where your perspective is important but you are not involved in group decision-making. The important point for this chapter is that this type of decision-making arises from a failure to form the group needed for collaboration and consensus.

Application Questions

Consider our example from the beginning of this chapter about deciding on a restaurant. Imagine it's Aunt Miriam's birthday, and your family is taking her out to dinner. She picks a steakhouse that is part of a national chain as the destination. What kind of decision-making is occurring? What are the pros and cons of her choice?

In the same situation, imagine that your brother recently became a vegetarian. You think that his options might be limited at the steakhouse. You decide to discuss some alternatives with Aunt Miriam. Who might be important to include in the discussion? Why?

You realize that other family members may also have preferences that would be important to include, so you ask who else wants to be involved in the decision. No one else expresses any preferences except your father, Aunt Miriam's brother, who wants to make sure that the destination is not too noisy. With all of these considerations, Aunt Miriam, your brother, your father, and you decide to try a new Thai place. When you mention this decision to your mother, she expresses the concern that Thai food disrupts your father's sleep. Which part of consensus decision-making does this input represent? In what ways might you integrate this new information into the group's decision-making? How does this example fit into our model of consensus decision-making?

Considering your current or desired role in healthcare, give examples of when you might engage in:

Individual decision-making

Group decision-making

Final Reflection Questions

Theodore Jackson is being evaluated for a kidney transplant. Both the medical and surgical kidney doctors believe a kidney transplant is appropriate. Who else should be involved in the decision to proceed with organ transplantation? If you were leading this group, how would you support the decision-making process around the decision to have Mr. Jackson receive a transplant? You may need to research which health professionals and other individuals make up this type of group.

During the group's discussion about Mr. Jackson's needs, everyone supports proceeding with kidney transplantation except for the nurse coordinator. This individual raises the concern of how Mr. Jackson will afford the expensive immunosuppressive medications after a transplant. How does this issue fit into our model of consensus decision-making? How might this concern be addressed?

All concerns are eventually resolved, and Mr. Jackson is scheduled for transplantation with a sibling as the donor. However, two days before the planned surgery, Mr. Jackson develops a fever. How might this information be integrated into our model of consensus decision-making? How might the group respond?

In your current or desired role in healthcare, think of an example of group decision-making. What are some strategies you might use to ensure that:

Your perspective is sought and integrated into decisions?

Colleagues' perspectives are sought and integrated into decisions?

Dissenting opinions are considered?

Optimal decisions are made for your patients?

Further Reading

A brief but thorough discussion of consensus decision-making can be found in *Rules for Reaching Consensus: A Modern Approach to Decision Making* (1994) by Steven Saint and James R. Lawson. This book may be more useful for leaders than for frontline healthcare practitioners, but it focuses on defining and addressing legitimate concerns as well as resolving conflict as we will discuss in chapter 11.

A slightly longer but similar book is *Consensus-Oriented Decision-Making: The CODM Model for Facilitating Groups to Widespread Agreement* (2011) by Tim Hartnett. This book includes more case studies, tables, and figures and focuses more on the relationships involved in consensus decision-making. For resolving conflict, it focuses on discussing concerns, finding a group answer, and empathizing with individuals who feel their concerns are not resolved.

Finally, I introduced the concept of psychological safety in this chapter. This is an important concept for groups and leaders of group. To read more on psychological safety in healthcare, start with "Making It Safe: The Effects of Leader Inclusiveness and Professional Status on Psychological Safety and Improvement Efforts in Health Care Teams" by Ingrid Nembhard and Amy Edmondson in *The Journal of Organizational Behavior* (2006).

CHAPTER 10

Hierarchy and Power

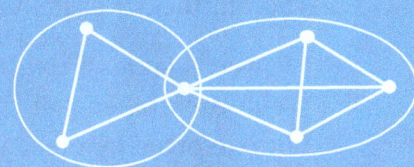

While we've referenced hierarchy throughout this book, it's time to take a deeper dive into understanding what hierarchy and the broader concept of power mean for collaboration. We're all very aware of the concept of power. From the time we are small children, we understand that some people have power, while others do not. But there are different types of power, and these types interact to shape both our relationships and our capacity to help our patients. Hierarchy is one way power becomes apparent.

The goal of this chapter is for you to develop a better understanding of power and recognize hierarchy as a manifestation of power. By the end of this chapter, you should be able to:

▶ define power,
▶ describe three types of power and give examples of each in healthcare, and
▶ give examples of the interplay between different types of power and how this interplay affects interprofessional practice and patient care.

Initial Reflection Questions

Think about someone you would think of as powerful in the public sphere—perhaps a politician or celebrity. Why is this person powerful? What gives this person influence over other people? (Often, powerful people have power for multiple reasons, so you may have several parts to your answer.)

Think about someone who has a lot of influence over you personally. It may a family member or friend. This influence represents a type of power. Why does this person have this power?

How does power differ between the two examples you gave above? Which person has more power relative to you as an individual? Why?

Power

For the purposes of this book, think about power as the ability to influence the behavior of other people. Someone with more capacity to influence others has more power, whereas someone with less capacity to influence others has less power. Let's explore this definition further by examining some qualities of power.

Important Qualities of Power:
• Socially constructed
• Relationship-dependent
• Variable symmetry
• Dynamic
• Grows and shrinks

Power is *socially constructed*, meaning that it is our relationships with each other that create power. While power can be enhanced or reinforced by other social structures, power begins with how we relate to each other. We give each other power. We'll examine how and why in a moment.

Power is *relationship-dependent*. Just because individuals have power in one relationship does not mean that they have power in other relationships. For example, I have a lot of power in my relationship with my school-aged children but less capacity to influence my parents. My children, who are completely spoiled by their grandparents, have a lot of power in relationship to their grandparents. You can think of our relationships as a triangle of power (see Figure 10.1). The relative amount of power depends on the relationship.

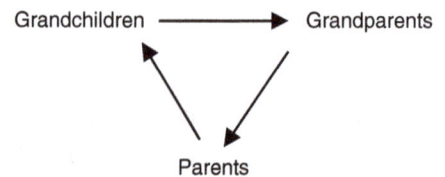

Figure 10.1 Power Within My Family With Arrows Showing Relative Influence. Source: Alan Dow

As this example also shows, power can have *variable symmetry*. If two people have a similar amount of power relative to each other, then power is symmetrical, but if their power toward each other differs, it is asymmetrical. Symmetrical power would seem to be better—after all, we want fair relationships with each other—but that's not necessarily true. For example, you probably don't want toddlers to have symmetrical power with their parents.

Power is *dynamic*. As children grow and become more independent, they have more power in relationship to their parents. As parents age and need more assistance from family, the children may have more power in those relationships. That's a dramatic, lifelong example, but power can also change from moment to moment as our relationships change, hence the term *power dynamics*.

Finally, total power can *grow and shrink*. A common mistake with power is to think of it as zero-sum, meaning that there is a fixed amount of power in the world or in your local environment. If power is zero-sum, then when one person gains more power, another person must have less power. But remember that power is socially constructed. We can give people more power—more influence over our behaviors—by developing trust, and they, in turn, can also give us more power. With respected colleagues, we want the total power—influence supported by trust—to be as high as possible. This point is really important for interprofessional practice, and we will come back to it.

Types of Power

Power comes in a number of types. While researchers have described power in many ways, for our purposes, I am going to focus on three main types of power: formal power, expert power, and relational power.

Formal Power

Formal power is the influence gained by having a position such as unit manager, department chair, or queen. When I described power as socially constructed, I noted that it can be reinforced or enhanced by social structures. Formal power is shaped greatly by social structures, especially the creation of hierarchy. Hierarchy is simply ranking people by power which, in turn, then creates relationships between people, usually leader-follower, that reinforce formal power.

When you think of hierarchy, you might first think of an organizational hierarchy with bosses and followers or a military hierarchy with generals, lieutenants, and privates. While hierarchies may be very clear in professional situations because of organizational charts, performance reviews, and status symbols like a general's star or a boss's corner office, that doesn't mean that hierarchy is absent in other places. Families and groups of friends can have more subtle hierarchies that define formal power in these relationships.

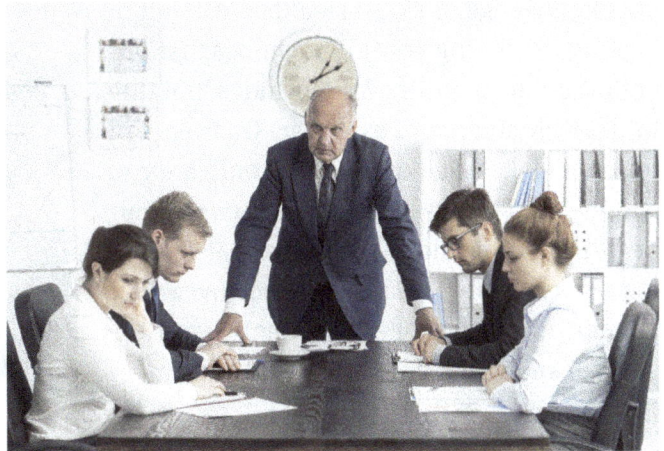

© Photographee.eu/Shutterstock.com

Being higher in the hierarchy usually means having access to significant tools that enhance formal power. These tools can be positive, like the ability to award a bonus, promote someone, or pass a student in a course, or they may be negative, like mandating a punishment, firing someone, or giving someone a lower grade. We, of course, want these tools used beneficently to help the group work better, and, thankfully, they usually are.

Because formal power depends on having a position, hierarchy may not seem socially constructed, but it is. Hierarchy remains because people, willfully or not, participate in it and recognize its value. Individuals can either support an existing hierarchy or work to undermine it. Supporting the hierarchy strengthens it while undermining the hierarchy is one way to advocate for change. This approach tends to slow down the group's work in healthcare, lead to dissatisfaction, and impact patients. Fortunately, there are usually better approaches to advocating for change, as we will see in chapter 13. Undermining the hierarchy can also have significant costs: you don't want to end up on the wrong end of a failed coup attempt.

Although hierarchy can be problematic, it is generally a good thing. We need people to be in charge. For one, it helps organize the work. Hierarchy establishes responsibilities and increases efficiency. In the planning phase, it determines leadership and the responsibility for ensuring that the group works effectively and fits within the larger environmental context. Hierarchy also provides pathways by which a group can acquire needed resources, like supplies or extra staffing.

However, we vary as individuals in our comfort with hierarchy, a concept called *power distance orientation*. Some people, whether they are low or high in a hierarchy, like being part of a hierarchical structure. It gives them a clear sense of where they stand, and they find that ranking reassuring. Other people chafe at hierarchy and would prefer that everyone interact as equals. Either extreme can be bad: you don't want people unquestioningly following orders, and you don't want people being unnecessarily disruptive. For our purposes, recognize that there is variation and that your power distance orientation may shape your comfort with hierarchy, your choice of professional roles, and how you and your colleagues interact.

Expert Power

Expert power is influence granted by specialized knowledge or skills. Healthcare is full of experts (including you!). Remember that our definition of a profession includes training to develop an area of expertise. Our years of training make us all experts. Not only are you gaining knowledge and skills through your healthcare education, but you are also gaining power. You will have influence over your patients and your colleagues due to your expertise, and that's not to be taken lightly.

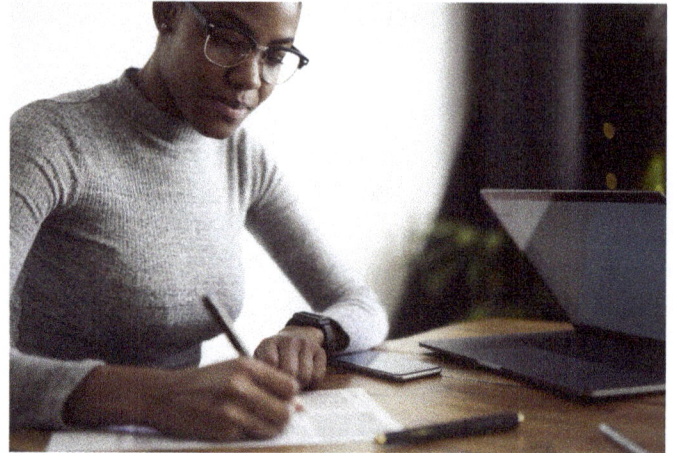

In many fields, formal power and expert power may not overlap. For example, in the basic science department of a university, while the best researchers often run large laboratories, they rarely ascend up the academic hierarchy to become deans or university presidents. These researchers' talents and aspirations do not align with ascending the institutional hierarchy to gain formal power. It's tough to win a Nobel Prize if you are stuck in administrative meetings all day.

Healthcare is different though. Expert healthcare practitioners often assume leadership roles because of their success as practitioners. The most common example occurs when successful physicians become hospital CEOs. This approach has two flaws. First, expertise as a practitioner and ability as an organizational leader do not necessarily overlap. Poor leadership abilities can hinder collaboration and overall effectiveness, which may lead practitioners to "work around" a formal leader.

Second, and more important for our purposes, depth of expertise within a profession is often equated with formal power. Physicians usually have the greatest depth of expertise in healthcare, at least as measured by years of training and riskiness of professional activities. This expert power has led to physicians, as a group, traditionally having the most formal power in healthcare. This disenfranchises all the other professions that bring their own valuable perspectives on how best to care for patients. While this has changed some over the past couple of decades (in part due to other professions establishing their own areas of deep expertise), physicians still remain the group with the most formal and expert power in healthcare.

Another group has gained increasing formal power in healthcare: administrators. As the structure of and payment for healthcare has become more complicated, the expertise of individuals with business training (expert power) has augmented the number and impact of administrative positions in organizations (formal power). This is necessary to manage modern healthcare but not clearly beneficial to overall health. Consider what kind of expertise you would most want leading healthcare—probably someone who understands patients more than billing though administrators are sensibly working to become better connected to patients.

© GaudiLab/Shutterstock.com

Finally, note that expert power developed through on-the-job experience can create an informal hierarchy. For example, a nurse who has 30 years of experience on a hospital ward has more expert power than a recent nursing school graduate, even if they both fill the same role within the hospital. The more junior nurse will defer to the more senior nurse such that the more senior nurse has expert power that supports formal power.

Relational Power

The final type of power we'll consider is *relational power*. Relational power is influence gained through trust and respect. In a way, it's the purest type of power because it does not depend on hierarchy or expertise. Everyone can have relational power. It's the easiest type of power to grow, but it's also very easy to lose. As our groups work toward becoming teams and developing their own norms, we are creating relational power.

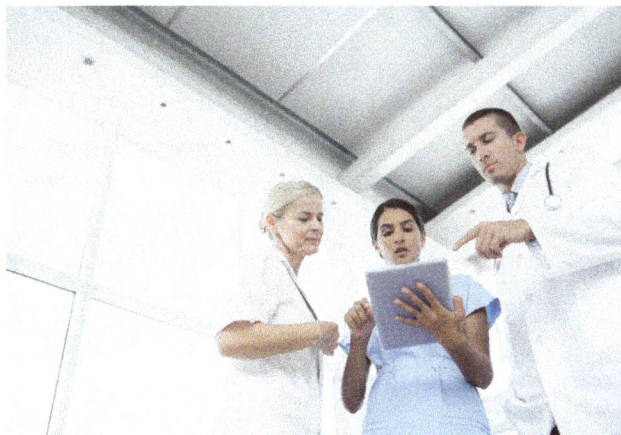
© wavebreakmedia/Shutterstock.com

Relational power interacts with formal power and expert power. As I have described relational power, someone you know may have come to your mind. If that person is a leader within your hierarchy or an expert, or both, he or she also has formal power and/or expert power. But it's that person's relational power that has left an imprint on you. Relational power is the most durable. When we give people relational power, we like them and trust their decisions.

The Types of Power and Group Formation

All three of these types of power are in action during interprofessional practice. Let's reexamine our prior exploration of group evolution and group process in the context of these types of power.

First, consider formal power. Individuals with formal power are identified as leaders. While people without formal power can become important leaders, those individuals positioned higher in the hierarchy are always and automatically designated as at least part of the leadership group. Someone else's abilities may make them better suited to being in charge, but formal power is rarely assigned by the group.

Because of this, formal power can create problems that lead to groups being stuck in the storming phase. The formal leader might not have the trust or respect of the group, possibly for good reason, and can clash with individuals with other types of power. In addition, different hierarchies can collide, leaving group members to figure out how these different representations for formal power fit together.

We will talk about how to navigate conflict in chapter 9, but the gist here is that formal power is important but not everything. In interprofessional practice, formal leaders are critical in the planning phase. They shape how groups interact by selecting group members, creating rules and policies, managing the overall process of group interaction, and providing access to resources. Formal leaders need to understand the broader context and how the group should interact with that context to, say, meet institutional goals or acquire necessary materials or expertise. But, as our groups form and storm, formal leaders need to support the leadership capacity of all of us. They should develop the leadership capacity of our entire group. Storming provides the space and time to clarify these leadership functions and, once we determine those roles, it's usually better for patients to stick with them rather than risk re-storming. This can be tricky business—being a good follower (see sidebar) is just as hard as being a good leader, especially when you don't get the same credit as the leader.

Followership

An important concept embedded in this discussion is *followership*. Followership is, in a sense, the opposite of leadership. It's the capacity or ability to be a good follower and let others lead. There are several reasons to be a good follower.

For one, you may not be experienced or expert enough to lead. That's pretty straightforward, but it helps us think about what it means for you to be a good follower: you defer to others who have power, fulfill your roles and responsibilities, provide input when you have something important to offer, and support morale. These are important tasks for any follower.

In the alternative, you might be too busy to lead. As your career unfolds, you will quickly find that you need to share leadership responsibilities. And, when that happens, you need to assume the role of a follower and act accordingly. For example, much of my job as an attending physician is to be a good follower for all the other practitioners around me. That can be a challenge, especially when you are a formal leader and are used to being responsible.

The other reason to act as a follower is when you are giving someone else experience as a leader. We do this all the time in academic medical centers. When I am rounding with a team of residents, I let the residents make almost all of the decisions. I might disagree with some of their decisions, but, unless another treatment decision has less risk or clear evidence of a greater benefit, I let the residents choose the course of action. I'm giving them autonomy to be leaders, and to do that, I have to be a good follower.

Related to this is another important part of being a follower: helping the leader lead. When a leader has deficiencies, a good follower helps the leader overcome those gaps so that the group can succeed. Instead of subverting the hierarchy, a follower can and should prod, suggest, assist, and support as needed. Leaders are made, not born; if you are a good follower, you make your leader better.

What about expert power in interprofessional groups? In the group formation phase, we need to make sure that we have the right expertise. As we move into the later phases, we may need to return to the team formation phase if we realize that we need additional expertise. In the storming and norming phases, expert power is also important. As we figure out how we fit together in a group, we grow to understand each other's areas of expertise and develop norms for combining that expertise to define professional responsibilities. These norms help us divide up work in the planning phase and address unexpected events during the action phase. We build our group's capacity to best leverage our expertise.

For example, some of my patients only speak Spanish. While my Spanish is passable, I avoid trying to speak Spanish to patients in the hospital so that neither side misses out on important information. Sometimes I work with translators over the phone, but my preference is to have a group member who speaks Spanish translate. That individual builds longitudinal rapport with the patient in a way that we lose when we only use the phone translators. Recognizing the expertise of Spanish proficiency in our group helps us develop new norms for working together and shapes our activities in the action phase ("Let's plan to all meet at 10 a.m. at the patient's room so we can see how he is doing.").

This brings us to relational power. Improving interprofessional practice, at least at the group level, depends in large part on increasing our relational power. As we move through the stages of group formation and begin performing, we are building relational power as we learn about each other, develop mutual trust, and share expertise and perspectives for how to approach work. Formal power and expert power underlie the work of groups, but it is relational power that determines whether the group will excel.

In addition, while all three types of power transfer from group to group, relational power may transfer the most. In a new or concurrent group, formal power and expert power stay the same—you tend to maintain both your place in the hierarchy and your level of expertise. But relational power grows. People who have worked together carry those relationships forward. Your reputation—hopefully a good one—precedes you.

Patients and Power

So far, we have not mentioned patients, but they are the essential people in healthcare. How does power affect them? With expert and formal power, patients have a strange inequity. While patients are the experts on themselves, they usually access health services seeking medical expertise. Practitioners have to integrate their health expertise with patients' preferences and perspectives as they co-develop recommendations. Similarly, there is a tension between the formal hierarchy of healthcare and a desire to give power to patients within the concept of patient-centeredness. We want patients to have authority over themselves, yet we care for them in a system with a strong hierarchy that treats them as outsiders. Patient expertise and patient-centeredness are important—yet so are the opinions of experts and the value of a set structure within the healthcare system. How do we resolve these tensions?

Relational power is the solution. It is the relationships we build with patients that help them and us navigate everyone's expertise, preferences, and hierarchy to best meet those patients' needs. Whether and how much the expertise and authority of a healthcare practitioner shapes a patient's care depends on the practitioner's personal connection to the patient. Patients want healthcare practitioners who are not just smart, self-assured, and revered by their colleagues; they also want practitioners who are compassionate and caring with them. At the end of the day, healthcare is about the quality of our relationships with our patients.

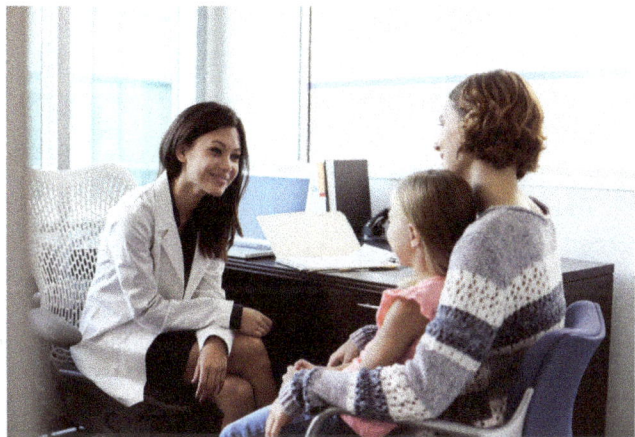

© Monkey Business Images/Shutterstock.com

Application Questions

Thinking about your role in your family, what are your sources of power in the following areas:

Formal power (your place in the hierarchy)

Expert power (your areas of expertise)

Relational power (your influence over others because of your relationships)

How do these different sources of power lead to an asymmetrical distribution of power?

Now, think about a specific role in your career, either in the present or future. In what ways is or will your work be affected by the following types of power:

Formal power

Expert power

Relational power

When will you be a follower, and when will you have opportunities to lead?

Final Reflection Questions

As mentioned in this chapter, formal power and expert power overlap more in healthcare than in most other fields. Do you think this is good or bad? Why or why not?

I described relational power as the solution to some of the power challenges in healthcare. Do you agree? How might our relationships help us with the other power challenges in healthcare?

This chapter discussed the importance of followership. Can you describe an example where you chose to be a follower even though you had the capacity to be a leader? What were the challenges, if any, of choosing to be a follower?

Further Reading

The psychologists John French and Bertram Raven first described five types of power in 1959. They later added a sixth type of power. These papers are still relevant today and worth reading if you want to expand beyond my simplified description above.

Deborah DiazGranados, Paul E. Mazmanian, Sheldon M. Retchin, and I discussed followership and delegation with a focus on medical residents in our 2013 *Academic Medicine* article, "Applying Organizational Science to Health Care: A Framework for Collaborative Practice."

A more in-depth discussion of followership can be found in "From Passive Recipients to Active Co-Producers— The Roles of Followers in the Leadership Process" published as part of the 2006 book *Follower-Centered Perspectives on Leadership: A Tribute to the Memory of James R. Meindl* by Boas Shamir, Rajnandini Pillai, Michelle C. Bligh, and Mary Uhl-Bien.

CHAPTER 11

Navigating Conflict

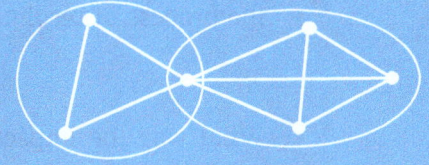

One of the most daunting parts of working with others is navigating conflict. While the main advantage of working with others is the diversity of expertise, abilities, and perspectives within a group, the main challenge is combining that diversity to reach the best decisions. Leading to those decisions are many small conflicts that we must first resolve.

This chapter builds on our understanding of group decision-making and power to explore how to approach conflict. By the end of this chapter, you will be able to:

▸ compare and contrast task conflict and interpersonal conflict,
▸ describe the relationship between the concept of position and the concept of intention,
▸ delineate a stepwise approach for navigating conflict,
▸ articulate the importance of external parties when navigating conflict, and
▸ describe how you might engage resistance to improve group function and resolve conflict.

Initial Reflection Questions

Think of a time where you disagreed with at least one other person on a course of action. It need not have been in a healthcare situation.

What was the position of each person involved in the disagreement? That is, what decision did each person want to reach?

For each of these people, what was the underlying intention or rationale for his or her position? Note: While it may be easy for you to articulate your own intention, it may be harder to articulate the intentions of others. Feel free to use your imagination, but it is important that you try to describe this intention as completely as you can.

Did intentions overlap in any areas? Were there areas where intentions were held more strongly by one person than others? Describe.

Was the conflict eventually resolved? If so, how? How did individuals' different intentions affect the process of resolution?

What was the impact of the conflict on the relationship(s) between the people involved in the conflict?

The Inevitability of Conflict

Most of us dread conflict, yet it is inevitable. Conflict is a basic function of life. It occurs across cultures and has even been noted in non-human animals. Successfully resolving many small conflicts is seen as essential for building friendships. Strange as it may seem, conflict may be what brings us together.

In healthcare, we encounter conflict all the time. Our work is complex and challenging, so the path forward is not always clear. We have differences of opinion, and we care about our patients and the outcomes

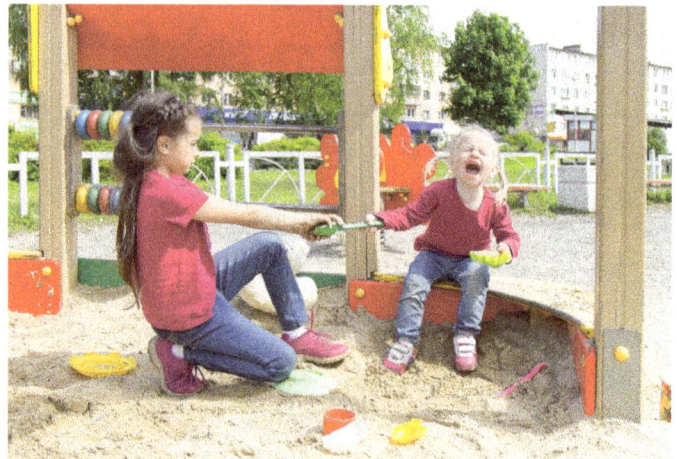
© Zabavna/Shutterstock.com

of our decisions. Conflict is often critical for finding the best path forward. And as much as we might like to avoid the stress of disagreements, conflict strengthens our identity as a person and a professional.

Sometimes conflict involves patients directly. While we will build on our group decision-making concepts here and keep patients to the side for the moment, note that conflict might be with the patient, not just around the patient. If the patient is involved in the conflict, he or she needs to be involved early in the process of navigating the conflict. We will return to the patient's role in conflict later; for now, the goal of this chapter is to help you navigate conflict to best move forward with the care of your patients while also building stronger relationships with your colleagues.

Two Types of Conflict

Conflict comes in two interrelated types: task conflict and interpersonal conflict. Differentiating between these two types is essential. *Task conflict* is conflict directly related to decisions about how to approach work. *Interpersonal conflict* is based on emotions and related to the relationships between the people involved in the work.

Task conflict can spark interpersonal conflict. As interpersonal conflict increases, the conflict becomes muddled with fear, anxiety, and uncertainty, which makes the underlying task conflict more challenging to resolve. Interpersonal conflict is normal, but you need to recognize and address it so that the group can address the task conflict at hand.

Aspirations for Conflict

Underlying conflict is the shared goal of reaching the best decision for our patients. We experience conflict because we care about those decisions. We are experts, and we have confidence in our individual opinion—which is a good thing. We also value collaboration and our shared commitment to making the best decisions for the patient based on everyone's perspectives. Let's take a moment to think about the characteristics of a "best decision." These characteristics can guide us when we are stuck in conflict.

Best decisions are **wise**. Based on the available information, they are the best possible choice. That does not mean that they will always be right. Sometimes we carefully consider all the available facts and yet still make a mistake. But we've been thoughtful and tried our best. Best decisions may be

> **Characteristics of Best Decisions:**
>
> - Wise
> - Efficient
> - Strengthen relationships

hard. Sometimes all options are lousy, yet we need to make a choice. What's important is that we make as careful a decision as possible.

Best decisions are **efficient**. We spend as much time as we need to make the decision and no longer. The world of healthcare is busy. We can't get bogged down with an inefficient decision-making process. We need to make decisions and move on to the rest of the work.

Best decisions **strengthen relationships**. Done well, making decisions with others builds trust and brings us closer together. Making decisions helps us norm and perform. We become a more collaborative group that is better at making decisions in the future. In contrast, if decision-making introduces interpersonal conflict that tears our group apart, even a wise, efficient decision can be a bad one.

Recognize the theme within all three of these characteristics—best decisions are defined by the process of reaching them, not the outcome. Sometimes these characteristics may seem in opposition—being wise seems slow and being efficient seems fast. That's why the process is important. We need to collaborate with our colleagues to decide how to balance wisdom and efficiency that builds relationships. If we are wise, if we proceed efficiently, and if we build our relationships throughout the decision-making process, we will reach the best decision we can and be better positioned to help our patients in the future.

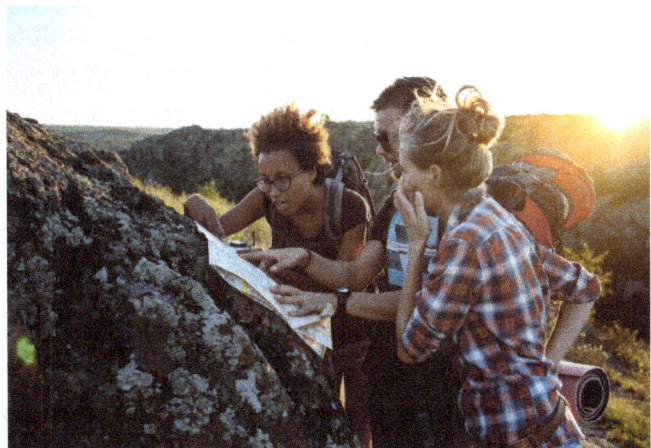

© Cookie Studio/Shutterstock.com

A Stepwise Approach to Resolving Conflict

Let's turn to the process of how to navigate conflict to reach the best decision. Here, I am providing a general framework that should be applicable across conflicts in healthcare and beyond. While many conflicts will not require the in-depth application of this framework, it offers an organized approach to fall back on when you need it. And the principles within transfer across all spheres of life.

You should see parallels between this information and the structure for group decision-making. The frameworks are similar, though this one goes deeper into difficult and emotionally charged situations while also bringing in some additional considerations. Here, the intermingled nature of interpersonal and task conflict is important, and the goal is for you to address both types of conflict as you step through the model. Think of it as advanced group decision-making.

Step 1: Affirm Relationships

As healthcare practitioners, our first instinct when faced with a conflict is to solve the problem. We are trained to analyze data, come up with a solution, and advocate for it. However, this is precisely the wrong way to approach conflict.

> **Steps in Conflict Resolution**
> - Affirm relationships
> - Define intentions
> - Develop solutions
> - Decide

We have conflict when our *position* differs from someone else's position. A position may be an approach to reach a goal. If our goal is to have a patient recover or help him or her stay healthy, we may have different positions about how best to do that. A position can also be a belief or attitude. Sometimes we may disagree about the best outcome—in other words, the goal itself is the area of conflict. When that happens, the goal becomes a position.

When we have competing positions, we need to resolve the conflict. But if we only focus on the positions, conflict resolution devolves into each person arguing for his or her position and against other people's position(s). We dig in because we are committed to our patients and confident in our abilities. Task conflict begets interpersonal conflict. Someone might "win" when the other side acquiesces, but the relationship is harmed. Decisions do not wisely leverage the expertise of the group, are not made efficiently, and do not strengthen relationships within the group. We won't reach the best decision.

Let's look at a different approach that begins with relationships. Before we can resolve task conflict, we need to resolve, or at least try to mitigate, interpersonal conflict. As we have seen, healthcare is a diverse, dynamic setting. We often work with new people who have different perspectives. As our groups constantly re-form and storm, the members of our current group may have limited experience with each other and may not have developed trust. Worse, group members may even carry animosity toward one another from prior interprofessional interactions where the effects of strong hierarchies and cultural traditions interfered with their ability to reach the best decisions. To set the stage to resolve conflict, we need to reaffirm the importance of our interprofessional collaboration and reinforce our shared approach to the care of the patient.

So, rather than immediately advocating for a position, the first step is to build relationships around our shared goals for the patient. Think of this as moving through storming and into norming. Why are we caring for this patient? What emotions are involved in providing this care? How are these emotions tangled up with the decisions that we need to make? Are we facing intertwined interpersonal and task conflict? If you're a leader—and anyone can be—your job is to listen and, less often, speak up to help the group evolve. To start, everyone needs to feel valued and to begin to build trust.

Step 2: Define Intentions

The next step in navigating conflict is to define *intentions*. Intentions are the expertise, values, hopes, and fears that underlie our positions. Some intentions may be based in our professional expertise, while others are part of who we are as a person.

By approaching conflict through intentions rather than arguing for positions, we view the situation at a more fundamental level. For example, when we affirmed the importance of our relationships and established that we all want to make the best decision for our patient, we defined an intention, one that is now shared. Now, we can build on that foundation to work toward a decision that we can all agree on.

Some questions can help us define our intentions. Thinking about our goals for the patient, what defines a good outcome? What aspects of patient care are important from your professional perspective? What is important to your colleagues in this situation? Most significantly, why are these aspects important to each person?

This process will define some areas where intentions agree or are at least compatible. In addition, it might define areas where intentions are incompatible. The goal for this step is to define the underlying intentions, determine areas of agreement, and identify important areas of disagreement. With any luck, the conflict may spontaneously resolve (see sidebar).

The Last Lemon

A grocery store manager came upon two customers arguing in the produce department. Only one lemon was left in the store, and both customers needed it. The first customer felt he had a claim to it because he saw it first. But, while he was retrieving a bag from the spool, the second customer reached over and grabbed the lemon. They began to argue and reached an impasse. How could the grocery store manager solve the problem?

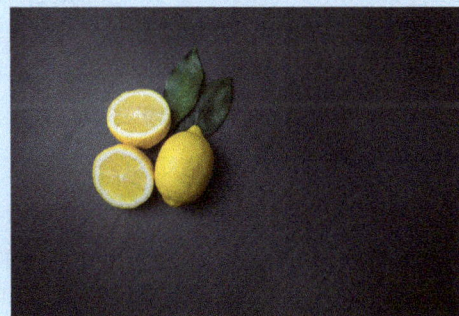

© paulkoo/Shutterstock.com

He did it by defining intentions. He asked why each customer needed the lemon. The first customer said, "I am baking a cake and need fresh lemon zest from the peel." The second customer replied, "I am making chicken piccata and need fresh lemon juice for the sauce." Grabbing a knife from the deli, the manager removed the peel from the lemon, gave it to the first customer, and gave the rest to the second customer. Both left happy, their underlying intentions having been met.

Think about what this means for how you expend your energy. Rather than fruitlessly advocating for your position, focus on defining everyone's intentions. Intentions are important manifestations of professional and personal identity. They build upon professional abilities, ethics, and personal characteristics. You should strive to define a compatible set of intentions that enhances the group's relationships and moves you toward your goal.

Step 3: Develop Possible Solutions

Presuming a solution has not magically appeared by this stage, it's time to consciously develop possible solutions based on our intentions and our shared goal for the patient. Start by having someone suggest a solution that attempts to reconcile the different intentions within the context of the goal for the patient. This initial solution is almost certain to be imperfect—if resolving conflict were easy, we wouldn't need this framework.

Now, the group can refine the proposed solution. Everyone should approach this solution with an open mind, considering how it might better meet our goal and stated intentions. The key behaviors involved here are providing and receiving criticism. Good criticism adds to and expands on the solution rather than suggesting an alternative. It's easy to throw cold water on an idea and end the discussion. What's much harder is to expand discussion and make a proposed solution better.

Similarly, whoever suggested the solution needs to be open to criticism. That person needs to embrace the imperfection of the original proposal and remain humble about making it better by integrating others' ideas. The goal here is to leverage the diversity of the group to discover the best decision. How can we learn from each other? How can we meet multiple intentions? Where can we find shared ideas that help us move ahead?

Once the initial solution has been fully explored, it may be necessary to identify and explore other solutions. Everyone should have an opportunity to propose additional solutions that the group refines in a similar process. Sometimes a solution that at first seems unpromising can, with the input of the group, become the best decision for that patient. In an ideal world, the goal is to fully explore a variety of solutions before moving into the final step.

Step 4: Decide

Finally, it's time to decide. It is important here to define objective criteria that stem from our intentions. You could think of defining objective criteria as a separate step, but the best time to complete that step can vary. These criteria can be developed during the earlier step of defining intentions, but that timing can hamper the exploratory work of developing solutions. Here, I am rolling them into our process of deciding.

Let's also bring in someone we haven't considered much yet—the patient. As we will discuss below, engaging patients in conflict depends on how central the patient is to the conflict. We should always provide patient-centered care, but conflict is not always centered on the patient. If we haven't involved the patient in resolving the conflict yet, now may be the time to bring the patient in to the conversation.

The group, possibly led by the patient, should consider what criteria should apply, their relative importance, and how we can assess them. While defining objective criteria can be challenging, this process is important. It helps us link our intentions to our possible solutions. Some questions, like "What will insurance pay for?", is a defining criterion for many decisions and of varying importance to different patients. Other criteria—like long-term prognosis or benefit—are unpredictable, but we must try our best. Defining criteria often establish norms that can be reused when making later decisions.

Once criteria are established, it's time to examine each possible solution based on the criteria. Like with consensus decision-making, the best decision may not be everyone's favorite solution, but it is one that everyone can live with. For a clinical decision, the patient has the final say, but it's important to try to incorporate everyone's values to ward off moral distress (see chapter 7). Applying criteria to possible solutions may also generate new ideas or new combinations of old ideas. That's fine—the goal is to make the best decision and get on with the rest of the work (see sidebar).

BATNA

BATNA or "Best Alternative to a Negotiated Agreement" is a key concept from negotiation that can help you navigate a decision. BATNA has implications both for group decision-making and resolving conflict in healthcare. Let's me give you some examples to describe the concept of BATNA.

Imagine that you are applying for jobs. If you have several suitable job offers, your BATNA is pretty good. If your first choice falls through, you have other options that are good alternatives. You are in a strong negotiating position.

However, if you only have one job offer, your BATNA isn't as strong. Without a backup plan, you need that job more. When you negotiate for that job, you have less leverage even if the employer doesn't know it.

Now, flip this situation around. The potential employer also has a BATNA. It may have several qualified candidates, or it may only have you. The more acceptable candidates the employer has, the stronger its BATNA, but if you're the only good candidate, their BATNA is lousy. In a negotiation, all sides have a BATNA, and you should try to figure out everyone's BATNA.

What about BATNA in healthcare? Usually, the BATNA is maintaining the status quo. If we can't agree, we continue the same approach which may have positives and negatives. BATNA becomes linked to the urgency for change. Sometimes we need to make an urgent decision because our BATNA isn't a very good option. Other times, we have less urgency because our BATNA is reasonable for the patient at the moment.

As you traverse conflict in healthcare, think about everyone's BATNA, especially the patient's. What are the advantages and disadvantages to not deciding and continuing the status quo? Sometimes the cost or risk associated with not deciding helps move people forward. For example, you might say, "We can talk about this more tomorrow, but I worry that we continue to expose this patient to the risk of a hospital-acquired infection." The patient's BATNA is something to keep in mind.

Failing to Decide

If the group fails to decide, it may be time to get help. Remember the characteristics of a best decision: wise, efficient, and supportive of relationships. By developing several solutions collaboratively, we have maximized the wisdom of the group and been supportive of relationships. But, if we have failed to decide, we need to maintain efficiency by getting help.

To get help in healthcare, you typically need to engage an external authority from the existing hierarchy. These leaders usually have the experience and perspective to help navigate challenging conflict. While this takes effort on their part, your work to date should make it easier. Your group has already created possible solutions and objective criteria that represent everyone's perspectives. These frame the issues for the external leader, who can guide your group about how to move forward, especially in those difficult situations centered on patients. Whatever their counsel, maintaining supportive relationships in your group is essential since you will almost certainly continue to collaborate with each other.

Channeling Resistance

Sometimes one colleague consistently opposes the rest of the group. This is a challenging situation, but there are approaches you can use to help navigate it. Some people have specific issues on which they have strong yet unconventional views. Other people simply like to be naysayers; it's their personality. And yet other people may be feeling the effects of burnout or stress in other areas of their lives. Regardless of the cause, working with and channeling resistance is necessary to moving the group forward. It also might lead to a better decision and build a stronger relationship between you and the resistant person. Usually these approaches work best in a one-to-one setting. They include:

1. **Define and explore the resistance.** Ask the resistant person to define his or her position. Although this alternative is unlikely to be accepted by the group at large, defining the position lets you explore the intentions behind it. For example, the resistant person may believe that a certain course is justified because of something that happened to a prior patient or based on some new evidence from the literature. Understanding their position might identify a way forward—perhaps even a better way.

2. **Consider the resistant person's criticism of the current plan.** If the group has otherwise reached consensus around a certain approach, create a venue to hear out the resistant person's criticism and try to understand the underlying intention. There may be something of merit that this person has struggled to express; he or she may just need time to think through this perspective. The goal is to make the best decision, and sometimes a resistor has identified an error in the group's decision-making process.

3. **Recognize that we work in a stressful environment.** The person who is resisting may just be frustrated. A cup of coffee or a kind ear may be the best approach. Think about who can take this person aside for a chat. Maybe the current area of conflict is not the real issue. We all bring our personal lives to work, and we all experience a lot of stress in our work. Sometimes we just need a friend to help us through.

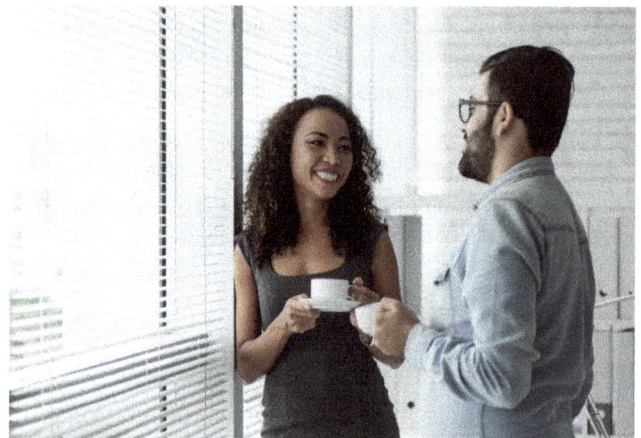

© Dragon Images/Shutterstock.com

Struggling with conflict is often associated with feeling less valued by the group, less secure in the group, and less compatible with the group. Someone who struggles with conflict deserves empathy and support. Though it may take more work up front, working through one incident of resistance can reduce future resistance and help this resistant person become a better collaborator.

Engaging Patients and Families in Conflict

Throughout this chapter, I have only tangentially referenced the role of patients and families. Integrating patients can be tricky and depends on the situation. Some conflicts arise strictly within the group of healthcare practitioners, while others directly involve patients. While the patient perspective is always important, when healthcare practitioners disagree, we might need to first work through our professional differences independent of the patient so that we can present him or her with a coherent plan. Because none of us individually has all the wisdom of the group, we usually need to combine our expertise prior to engaging patients to streamline decision-making.

That being said, you should always think about how the patient relates to the conflict. If the patient is central to the conflict, he or she needs to be involved from the beginning: affirming relationships and goals, defining intentions, developing solutions, and deciding. In addition, recognize that for the most challenging situations, we will all be uncertain. Maintaining a focus on the patient can support a dialogue that enables us all to find the best decision (see sidebar).

Going Home

When I was newly practicing, one young patient taught me a lot about collaborating with families and colleagues. He had been in a horrific car crash and suffered a significant brain injury. By the time I became involved in his care, he had already been in the hospital for over six months. Over several weeks, I watched him regain some capacity to use his hands and answer questions with simple words, but he was not walking or feeding himself. While the prognosis for a complete neurological recovery was grim, he was doing well enough that he could soon leave the hospital. This presented a problem.

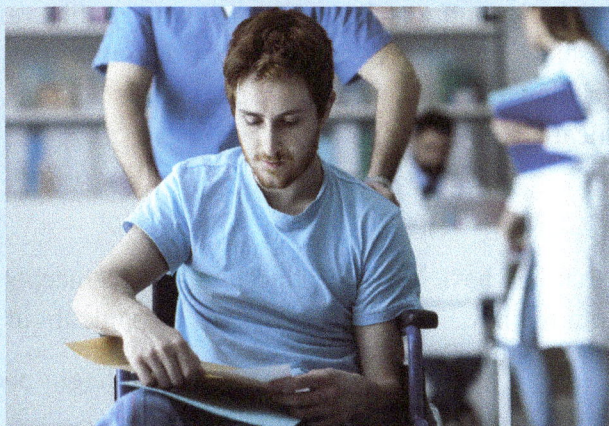

© Sotck-Asso/Shutterstock.com

The only real option he had was to go home with his brother. They lived together before the crash, and his brother occasionally visited him in the hospital. The patient had no other family in the area. In addition, he was not insured. He was not a U.S. citizen, so he did not qualify for Medicaid to pay for ongoing care in a nursing home. Returning to his shared home with his brother was the only feasible option.

His brother was understandably hesitant. He worried about providing ongoing care for the patient. He was concerned about how much everything would cost. He was apprehensive about how the obligations of caring for his brother would shape his own life. Most of all, he wanted to make the right decision for his brother, and none of the options were clearly the best.

Through a series of conversations with his brother, the hospital's care coordinators, and our group of frontline practitioners (including nurses, a nurse practitioner, a pharmacist, physicians, a physical therapist, an occupational therapist, a speech therapist, and a social worker), we created a plan. First, we emphasized our goals and intentions of wanting the best for the patient. We would make sure that he had access to practitioners for continued rehabilitation and follow-up care, and he could always come back to the hospital if his condition worsened. Building trust with the patient's brother was essential. I gave him my direct contact information in case an emergency, or even just uncertainty, arose.

Then, we built on everyone's intentions to work out what kind of support he would need at home, both from the brother's point of view and the perspective of the various practitioners. Some of this support was expensive, such as intensive in-home care. While the care coordinators initially balked at paying for this care, when we compared it to the cost of keeping him in the hospital, they arranged to have the hospital support the additional care in order to meet our shared intentions and goal. Finally, after weeks of work and months of hospitalization, we had a plan, and the patient went home with his brother.

The first couple of days after he left the hospital, all of us were anxious. Various practitioners heard from the patient's brother about a variety of concerns. As a group of healthcare practitioners, we kept each other in the loop.

Then it became quiet. Other than an occasional order I had to sign from the home health agency or an update from when someone called to check in with the brother, we heard little. About a month later, the patient was briefly readmitted with a fever, but he quickly got better and went back home.

About a year passed with little communication. I wondered whether something bad had happened to the patient or whether he had ended up in another hospital.

Then, one day, I was walking down the street outside my hospital when someone flagged me down on the sidewalk. It was the patient's brother—and walking next to him was the patient. While the patient was still debilitated, he was walking with assistance and he could speak haltingly. As they both profusely thanked me for my help, I marveled at his recovery. Navigating difficult decisions is never easy, but, in this case, the patient, his brother, and our group of practitioners had success.

Conflict Beyond Healthcare

Because you resolve conflict all the time, much of this chapter may have resonated with your own personal experience. What's important is that you have a way to think through conflict so that you can navigate it successfully in novel situations. This goal of this chapter was to give you a stepwise framework and some terminology to describe the process of resolving conflict. Life gives us plenty of opportunities to practice.

As you think about conflict, recognize how conflict resolution is engrained in rituals to help us identify, discuss, and resolve conflict. Just remember, it's not about winning. No one wins a marriage or a relationship with a sibling or parent. It's about making shared decisions that work for all of us. Healthcare is no different.

Application Questions

Now that you have been introduced to some concepts for navigating conflict, reexamine your example from the initial reflection questions to think about what you might have done differently.

How might you better have understood different people's intentions? Their BATNAs?

How might you have better developed possible solutions?

How might you have reached a better decision? What criteria might you have used?

In this chapter, I noted that conflict involving a patient is different than conflict around a patient. Looking at our stepwise approach, what are some key differences between these two types of conflict?

Final Reflection Questions

Can you think of an example when conflict ultimately strengthened a relationship? If so, describe it.

If you need an external party to help resolve a conflict, what characteristics of an external party would make that person good at resolving this conflict? How would you approach this person? How can you make the most of this interaction?

Try to identify a time when you were involved in conflict within a group where you felt poorly integrated. How did you feel about the process of conflict? Did you feel resistant or disengaged? What was the result of the conflict? How did you feel about the resolution? What lessons, if any, can you learn from this incident?

Further Reading

The most famous book about resolving conflict is *Getting to Yes*, written by William Ury and Roger Fisher in 1981. The material in this book was the source for much of this chapter. If you want to explore these concepts more deeply and with more examples, this book is worth reading.

Natural Conflict Resolution, a book compiled by Filippo Aureli and Frans de Waal in 2000, is a collection of chapters by various authors examining conflict from many perspectives. While much of this book focuses on conflict between non-human primates and other mammals, the chapters are a good starting point to read more about conflict resolution. The framework in chapter 16 and the final chapter are particularly useful.

CHAPTER 12

Giving and Receiving Feedback

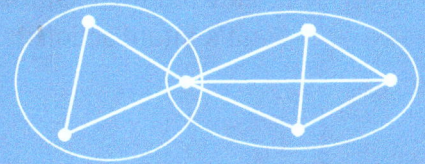

Receiving feedback is the primary means by which both individuals and groups can improve. Yet, despite its importance, we aren't very good at receiving critical feedback and even worse and giving helpful feedback. Feedback inspires many emotions, can be difficult to interpret correctly, and may not lead to appropriate changes.

To help with these challenges, in this chapter, we will look at some simple tips to improve the process of giving and receiving feedback. By the end of this chapter, you should be able to:

- identify how best to receive feedback to lead to positive change,
- describe how to give feedback to help someone else improve,
- compare and contrast approaches for multi-source feedback with interpersonal feedback, and
- recognize the value of a strengths-based approach for feedback.

Initial Reflection Questions

Think about a time when you received feedback. The more challenging the feedback, the better.

What emotions did you feel around the process of receiving feedback? How did those emotions affect the way you received the feedback?

Do you feel like you fully understood the feedback at the time, or were there gaps in your understanding? If there were gaps, why?

How did you change your future actions in response to the feedback? What, if anything, about those changes was challenging?

Think about a time when you gave feedback.

Did you feel confident and comfortable in your approach to giving feedback? Why or why not?

How did the recipient respond to the feedback you gave? Was it effective in changing the recipient's future actions?

Feedback

Feedback is essential for improving. The research is clear: people who receive feedback get better at all sorts of activities more quickly than people who do not receive feedback. But receiving feedback is not just a simple checkbox. The quality of the feedback and how the receivers integrate that feedback into their future performance also matter. Handling feedback well is one of the most important tools we have for improving our collective performance.

There are a number of ways to get feedback: in person, in a written performance review, or sometimes even through the grapevine. In this chapter, we are mainly focusing on direct, one-to-one, interpersonal feedback. Because this book focuses on collaboration and interpersonal relationships, this is the type of feedback most relevant to us here. We are most likely to use interpersonal feedback as we transition from the action phase to the planning phase of group work, review with someone his or her role in a consensus decision-making process, or deconstruct a time of storming and conflict.

We may also use feedback in other ways relevant to interprofessional practice. An example is multisource or 360-degree feedback. In this method, a number of people provide feedback about one group member; the feedback is then anonymized, aggregated, and shared with the receiver. Since this approach is increasingly popular, I will touch on it briefly and discuss how our principles of interpersonal feedback integrate with the process of multisource feedback.

Receiving Feedback

Let's start with receiving feedback since that will help us think empathetically about giving feedback. Receiving feedback is hard. It can provoke strong emotions—fear, sadness, anger, disappointment—and defensiveness. Those responses are normal, but they can also interfere with us making the most from the feedback. So, let's look at a stepwise approach to help us receive feedback and use it to improve our performance.

First, embrace the emotions involved with feedback. Not only does the receiver of the feedback have an emotional response, but also the giver of the feedback feels emotions around the feedback. Providing feedback takes effort, and the giver is putting in energy. In addition, the giver is taking a risk. No one wants to be the brunt of the receiver's anger, tears,

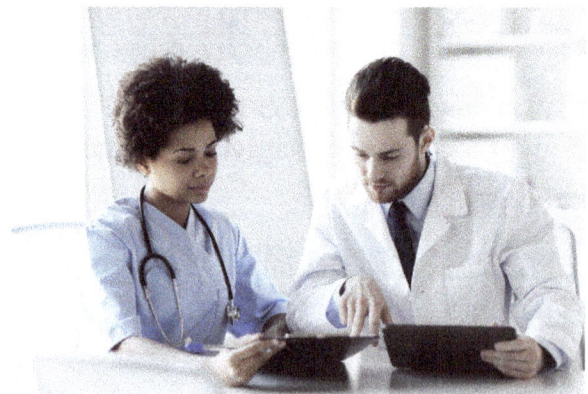

© Syda Productions/Shutterstock.com

Tasks in Receiving Feedback

1. Reconcile emotions
2. Understand meaning
3. Identify changes

or disappointment. If you are receiving critical feedback, recognize that the giver of that feedback cares about your performance and wants to help you.

Your first task when receiving feedback is to help the giver by trying not to let your emotions get in the way of understanding the message in the feedback. Recognize your emotional reaction and don't let it hinder the rest of the feedback conversation. You might feel all sorts of things, and those emotions are valid, but you need to put them aside for the moment. (This is a central precept of the mindfulness movement that is being used to help practitioners navigate stress and burnout in the challenging environment of healthcare.) After the feedback conversation, you can work through your emotions with friends, family, other colleagues, or possibly even the giver. Just don't let your feelings sidetrack the feedback conversation.

Your second task is to try to understand the feedback. Good feedback is specific and actionable; you know exactly how to change after receiving it. However, you're not always going to get "good" feedback. It can be difficult to give good feedback, particularly when the giver is not sure of the best way for you to improve your performance. This is particularly true in the complex interprofessional world of healthcare. Therefore, it's your job to try to understand what is driving the feedback, so you can identify for yourself how to improve.

To help you with this task, I encourage you to be curious and humble. Something has provoked the feedback. It's possible that an event, or your behavior within it, was misconstrued or misunderstood. Or, potentially, there is some truth there, and you have yet to recognize it. We all have blind spots. Be open and receptive as you try to understand what is driving the feedback and what the implications are for you. Ask lots of questions, and listen more than you talk.

The third and final task is to translate the feedback into specific changes in your behavior. This process can be thought of as meaning-making, where you take your understanding of the feedback and incorporate it into the way you do your professional activities. Take time to reflect on the feedback and determine how it should shape your approach to work. Circling back with the person who provided the feedback or discussing it with other colleagues can be a useful way to make sure that you understood the feedback correctly and that you're changing in a reasonable way. This clarification also helps to build rapport with others in your group as those people help you succeed. Feedback is precious, and only you can make the most of it.

Receiving Multisource Feedback

With multisource feedback, the concept of how to receive feedback is similar, though the process can be more challenging. Under this approach, you might receive a compiled set of ratings and comments. Maybe you will be compared to some benchmark or to the rest of the group. Typically, you won't have a designated person to discuss the feedback with or, if you do, that person will not have insights into the specific underlying intentions of the feedback. You're more on your own to understand the feedback, though it can be very rich.

However, your process for interpreting feedback should be similar. First, check your emotions: the two biggest mistakes in receiving feedback are blowing it off or taking it too seriously. You've got to try to find the middle ground. A good example is faculty getting student course evaluations. I always read mine at least twice: the first time to get defensive, angry, and disappointed and the second time to actually identify the substance that will help me improve.

Next, try to find the meaning in the feedback. You may need to solicit help from colleagues to get their impressions. Try to pick colleagues who won't sugarcoat their opinions. It can actually be better to pick someone you respect but don't know well. You can build a relationship (interprofessionally!) while getting a valuable outside perspective on the feedback. Your overall goal remains the same: to figure out whether and how to change your behavior in response to the feedback so you can be a better member of the group. You'll likely be getting multisource feedback again soon so you can see how much of a difference your adjustments made.

Giving Feedback

Now that we've examined receiving feedback, let's look at giving feedback with the same lens. While you may have had many opportunities to receive feedback, you may not have given lots of feedback, especially if you are a student. While anonymous evaluations of courses and professors are commonly used in education, giving great feedback depends on having an interpersonal relationship.

Tasks in Giving Feedback
1. Plan for and address emotions
2. Strive for clarity
3. Manage the reaction
4. Respond to questions
5. Decide on change

As we've discussed, feedback conversations inspire many potential emotions, including your own as the giver. Almost always, you will be giving feedback because you want the other person to improve. (In this book, we will not cover remediation conversations where you are functioning as an authority figure and telling someone to either improve or else.) Even though your heart is in the right place, you may feel trepidation about the conversation. The receiver will also certainly have concerns, right from the moment that you schedule the conversation. Fear is normal when someone says, "I'd like to give you some feedback."

How do we handle these emotions? First, pat yourself on the back for giving someone feedback. It's hard, and you are doing it because you care about the receiver and your work together. Embrace that. Not only will it steel your resolve, but it will also help you frame the feedback conversation by explicitly saying where you are coming from. The receiver needs the reassurance!

In addition, plan where and when you have the conversation. You want privacy and quiet—not always the easiest things to find in healthcare, but do your best. Later in a shift is usually better than the more hectic start of the day. Think about whether you need Kleenex, some water, or anything else. You might want someone else with you, but generally this just raises the stakes of the conversation and could muddy the waters of your feedback.

Your second task in giving feedback is to give the feedback as clearly as possible. You might think you are well-informed about whatever is driving this feedback conversation, but it's a good idea to talk with other people ahead of time to make sure that you fully understand the issues. You may find that you think differently about these issues than your colleagues do. If you don't have these conversations in advance, your feedback may be incomplete or erroneous. It's helpful to be able to represent the perspective of the group, and that can take some planning. By developing clarity about your feedback and its intent, you'll have a better chance of clearly communicating feedback that is specific and useful.

Your third task is managing the receiver's reaction to the feedback. When we hear challenging information about ourselves, all of us do similar things: we deny, we explain, we get angry or sad. This is normal, and your job as the giver of the feedback is to be patient and listen. Stay firm and clarify the meaning of the feedback as needed, but avoid arguing or backing down. You can see why it's important to both understand and convey the intent of the feedback here.

At this point, you've got a decision to make. Usually, you can weather the emotions around the feedback and move on to the next step. But it's okay to pause the conversation here if the reaction remains emotional. If the receiver isn't ready to proceed in the conversation, you'd be wise to plan to meet again later.

Your fourth task—whenever it occurs—is to respond to the receiver's questions. Hopefully, people who receive feedback will want to explore what you said and co-construct with you what it means for them and how their behaviors should change. Give the receiver space and time to process and reflect. You don't have to finish this step all at once during the initial feedback conversation, but you will want to be available for further discussions. The goal is to start a conversation about whatever the area of concern is and help the receiver work to improve.

Finally, your last task is to ensure that your response to questions helps lead the receiver to make lasting change. Realize that the solution may not be individual: it may depend on overall changes to the group or the system. You've invested in this receiver so far, and now you may need to continue to invest more to implement and sustain change, either by supporting the receiver as an individual or by developing a broader effort across the group. Be proud of yourself for your commitment to effect change. Hopefully, the receiver will acknowledge and appreciate it someday.

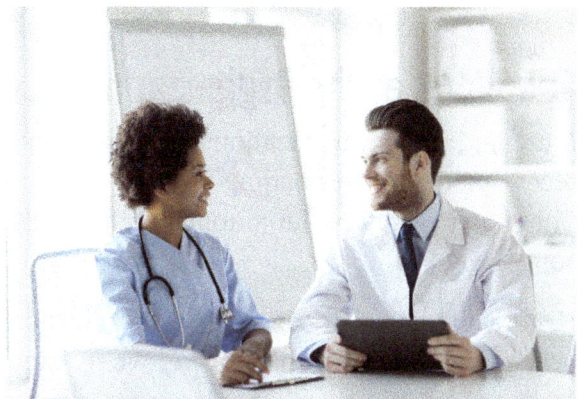

© Syda Productions/Shutterstock.com

Giving Multisource Feedback

You will also have many opportunities to contribute to group feedback that will be given to someone else. This person may be a peer, supervisor, faculty member, or trainee. This type of feedback also takes effort, but it's applied in a different way. When giving multisource feedback, you really have to pay attention to others' behaviors. Recognize when the time for feedback is coming up so you can keep your eyes peeled.

When you provide feedback, your job is to provide comments that are clear and actionable. One way to think about it is to assess whether your comments would be useful to you if you received them. In some settings, you have a choice to make about how anonymous you want your comments to be. On the one hand, you may want to keep your identity secret and let the overall group drive change. On the other hand, identifying yourself in the feedback could help the group more by giving the receiver more specific information and possibly triggering an important, relationship-building conversation with you about your feedback. If you decide to identify yourself, remember to think about how you can frame your feedback as coming from a place of good intentions and a desire to help that person.

One more consideration about feedback: many studies have shown biases based on gender, race, profession, and other characteristics in how feedback is both given and received. That's way too deep a subject to cover here, but think objectively about whether you are unintentionally introducing bias into your feedback based on these characteristics. Most people are.

> **The Feedback Sandwich**
>
> One popular technique for teaching about feedback is the feedback sandwich. It's a tactic that reinforces the concepts we discussed above and a useful way to think about integrating them in practice. During the feedback sandwich, the giver provides positive feedback (the bottom layer of bread), then negative feedback (the "meat"), before closing with more positive feedback (the top layer of bread). Let's apply our concepts above to this model:
>
> - The bottom layer of bread is really setting the stage for the meat. The giver is showing investment in the receiver and indicating that this conversation is a safe space. It's setting the stage for the meat.
> - The meat is the clear and actionable feedback. Here's what you really want to say.
> - The top layer of bread demonstrates ongoing support of the receiver. It maintains rapport and reassures the receiver of the giver's commitment and concern.
>
> I tend not to use this model and have felt it to be awkward when people have used it on me, but it is a good cognitive aid to help you when you are first giving feedback. Realize that the feedback sandwich does not necessarily help either the giver or the receiver identify future changes. Also, it can kind of whip the receiver around from positive to negative and back to positive. Think of it as feedback with training wheels and, as you get more practice, develop your own conversational approach based on the underlying feedback tasks.

Feedback at the Organizational Level

More and more, organizations are beginning to think about their areas of concern differently. One recent model for responding to areas of concern at the organizational level is *appreciative inquiry*. These models are useful to touch on and help us think another way about feedback at the interpersonal level.

Historically, areas of concerns in organizations were looked at as problems to be solved. This feels very familiar to us in healthcare; we're fixers. However, this approach oversimplifies problems in complex organizations. Problems are quickly fixed with short-term success, but the underlying causes are neither identified nor changed. The system continues to have weaknesses, and solutions are patchwork and inadequate.

In contrast, appreciative inquiry looks at areas of concerns not as problems to be solved but as mysteries to be embraced. Under appreciative inquiry, the process of examining areas of concerns is used to build stronger collaboration, increase team leadership, and solidify organizations. You can see the similarities to how we think about the benefits of interprofessional practice.

Let's briefly examine one approach from appreciative inquiry and think about the implications for interpersonal feedback. Appreciative inquiry is a strengths-based approach, meaning the focus is not on problems and deficiencies but rather on what do we do well and how can we leverage those positives to address an area of concern.

The first step of appreciative inquiry is to define the area of concern. However, instead of thinking of this area of concern as a problem, it should be seen as a result of a complex system. Defining the area of concern should also include identifying the positive aspects of the area and the strengths that surround it. In some ways, you can think about this as identifying potential and assessing available resources.

The second step involves defining perspectives and themes. Again, we are trying to identify strengths and positives. You can imagine that if we are trying to improve a struggling clinical unit, we might identify a positive of commitment to patients or high levels of camaraderie among nursing assistants. Here, we are refining and adding to our work from the first step to think about bolstering the system.

The third step is to describe the desired future. Here, the stories, themes, and strengths we've identified inspire us to think about what the area of concern could become. We start to see how our positives can be the foundation for a better future. This step is aspirational and leads us to dream about big changes.

Finally, the last step is to develop the innovations needed to reach the desired future. Here is where dreams get converted to pragmatic next steps. Plans are put in place to help everyone reach their goals. The goal is solutions that prevent the weaknesses in the system that lead to the area of concern.

Recognize how these principles fit with our model for individual feedback. In step one, you define the area of concern based on feedback, but you do that in relationship to the individual's and the clinical unit's strengths. From that definition, you can collaborate with the receiver and colleagues to further explore those strengths and think about how things could be based on those strengths. Finally, your group decides on steps that will help it reach the future.

Consider the example of an inpatient care partner who does not having time to turn a disabled patient every 30 minutes. Let's imagine that care partner has multiple, time-sensitive responsibilities and is very conscientious about feeding and bathing patients thoroughly. She gets caught up in that work and misses some of the turning responsibilities. Based on these strengths, a pragmatic, strengths-based solution would be to have the care partner focus on bathing and feeding additional patients and have another practitioner take on the responsibility of turning patients. Rather than seeing the missed turns as a deficiency, they define an opportunity to reconsider the work on the unit and build on the practitioners' strengths to provide better care for all the patients.

While this approach is just one way to think about feedback, it transforms the feedback conversation from a negative-leaning discussion of remediation to an inspirational conversation that engages the broader group to think about overall improvements to their work. By focusing on strengths and positives rather than harping on negative aspects, we may find better solutions to our challenges.

Humility

While I touched on this before, it bears repeating: above all, approach feedback with humility. Whether you are giving or receiving feedback, you are likely to learn something you didn't know, a perspective you had not considered, something about someone you didn't know, or an idea that will dramatically improve the care of your patients. Feedback conversations are about interaction. They are a great opportunity for all of us to learn and build stronger relationships with each other. And the key to that is engaging in them with humility.

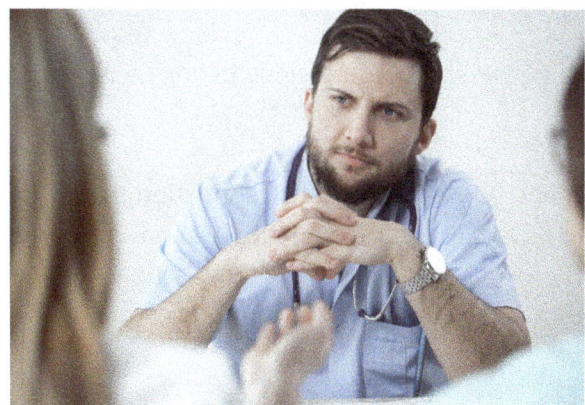

© Photographee.eu/Shutterstock.com

Application Questions

Think about someone you'd like to give feedback to. This could be a colleague, peer, family member, or someone else.

What is the content of the feedback? How would you provide it in a clear and actionable way? Who else might help you clarify the feedback, and how could you communicate with that person before the conversation?

Where and how would you plan the feedback conversation to show your support of the person and help reconcile emotions?

What kind of reaction do you anticipate from your feedback? How might you handle that situation?

Final Reflection Questions

Now that we've analyzed feedback, think about a prior conversation where you received feedback. It can be the example from the start of the chapter or a different example.

How well did the giver do at providing you with feedback? Did he or she help you identify and manage your emotions? Was this person clear in the feedback so that you understood his or her intentions? Did this person help you make and sustain change?

How well did you manage your emotions? What did you feel, and did your feelings interfere with your ability to process the feedback? Did you do anything to help yourself manage your emotions after you received the feedback?

Did you successfully change in response to the feedback? Why or why not?

The diversity of professions in healthcare can both hinder and help feedback. Why? Give examples.

Think about your prior participation in providing multisource feedback. Course and faculty evaluations are an example from education, but you may also have a workplace-based example. How could you do a better job of providing feedback in these venues? What is challenging about providing better feedback through this method?

If you have received, multi-source feedback, describe you reactions. What was you initial reaction? What about later? Did you make changes based on this feedback? Why or why not?

Further Reading

Appreciative Inquiry: Change at the Speed of Imagination (2010) by Jane Magruder Watkins, Bernard Mohr, and Ralph Kelly describes how the appreciative inquiry technique can be applied to changing an organization. If you are interested in this concept and want to read about broader applications as well as the history of this field and some case studies, this book is a good place to start.

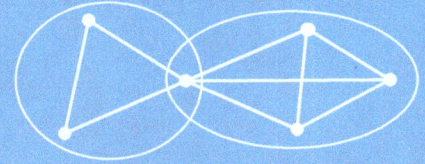

Even if you engage in flawless interprofessional collaboration with your colleagues, you can't solve all the challenges in healthcare. As we saw in chapter 6, factors at the organizational and societal levels shape our patients' lives and the ways that we collaborate. One way to influence organizational drivers of collaboration is by advocating up the traditional hierarchy. In this approach, we can identify frontline problems, bring them to our leaders' attention, and get support to implement change.

The purpose of this chapter is to equip you with the skills you need to advocate for change at the organizational level. While you may not be a decision-maker at the level of your organization or society at large, you can nonetheless advocate for decisions that you want to see made. And these skills are useful in other contexts as well: you can apply them outside your organization for societal change, and you may find them useful as you navigate conflict and work to collaborate better.

By the end of this chapter, you will be able to:

▸ define advocacy and explain its role in enhancing interprofessional practice,
▸ outline the characteristics of an advocacy goal that is likely to be successful,
▸ describe some strategies to increase the likelihood of successful advocacy, and
▸ identify why interprofessional advocacy is important.

Initial Reflection Questions

Think of a time when you advocated for something, ideally when you advocated for your position to someone with more authority. Work-based examples would be best, but you could also use an example from school or with your parents when you were younger. Think about the following questions.

What was your ultimate goal? Think about your intentions as we defined them when we discussed conflict in chapter 11.

Were there intermediate steps to your goal? If so, what were they?

What strategies did you use to advocate for your goal?

What was the end result? Did any of your strategies work better than others? Why or why not?

Defining Advocacy

Advocacy is the process of seeking broader or more influential support for a position. For our purposes, we will frame advocacy as trying to influence decisions within your organization to enhance your work and your patients' outcomes. While you can advocate to many parties—patients, their families, colleagues, policymakers, governmental officials, and others—here we are focusing on advocating to leaders within your organization. You can also advocate for many goals, but our focus is on improving collaboration and your patients' outcomes. However, advocacy principles are similar, regardless of the audience or goal. I encourage you to apply these principles elsewhere and to learn more about advocacy, especially political advocacy, if it interests you.

Advocacy gives voice to a problem and usually proposes a solution. For example, because our patients receive imperfect health services, they can usually identify ways that care could be improved. Yet, they rarely have avenues to voice their concerns and ideas. Advocacy is an approach to help them raise awareness of these problems and solutions.

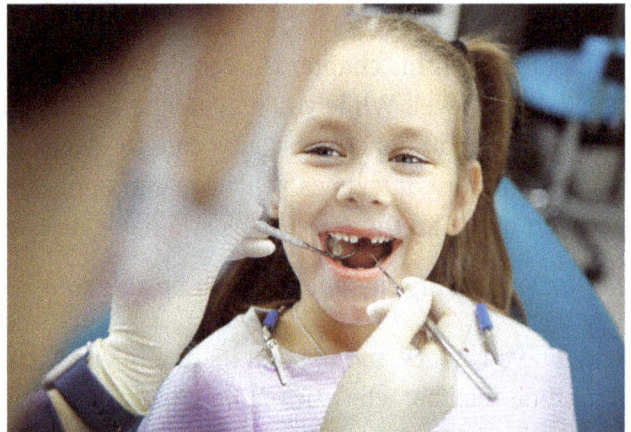

© i121/Shutterstock.com

Similarly, as frontline healthcare practitioners, we frequently recognize areas where care could be improved. And because we are experts in our practice, we often have insights about solutions to these problems that might be feasible. But how often do we voice these ideas to leadership?

Take medical error reporting. Less than 10 percent of medical errors in hospitals are reported. Some professions (such as nursing) are better than others (such as physicians), but none are exceptional. When asked why they don't report errors, practitioners cite a number of reasons. The two most common reasons are time constraints and a belief that nothing will be done about the problem. In other words, practitioners don't make it a priority to voice their concerns because they don't feel empowered to create change. Clearly, we need to learn to be advocates.

My hope for you is that you recognize your role as an advocate. As a frontline leader, you should advocate for what you need to improve the care of your patients. As you do so, you will gain power through relational and, eventually, formal mechanisms. If you want to make a difference in the system, diligent and consistent advocacy is the first step toward gaining that influence.

Defining a Problem for Advocacy

Problems in healthcare, especially the problems worth solving, are complex. If the solutions were easy, the problems would already be solved. Because of this complexity, our first step is to clearly define the problem that we will advocate about. This step is the foundation for the other steps in advocacy.

Bounded Problems	Unbounded Problems
Discrete	ill-defined
Time-limited	Boundaryless
Specific	Fuzzy
Solutions come to mind	Seem unsolvable

Figure 13.1 A Comparison of Bounded and Unbounded Problems. Source: Alan Dow based on the work of Watson and Watson (1986).

Defining a solvable problems in a complex system is not easy. An important concept is that problems can be either bounded or unbounded (see figure 13.1).

Bounded problems are discrete. You can describe them in detail. As you describe them, you can place limits around them to specific locations or times. For bounded problems, you should be able to think of some possible solutions though it may not be clear which solution is best.

In contrast, unbounded problems are ill-defined. They spread across many different settings and lack a definite conclusion or timeline. Unbounded problems seem to defy solutions.

While we can't ignore unbounded problems, to advocate successfully and ultimately implement change, we need to find a bounded problem. For example, healthcare inequalities are an unbounded problem. They are real and important issues that we need to solve. But it is challenging to identify specific solutions that would solve all health inequalities at once. These inequalities occur across different settings and seem unsolvable.

In comparison, a specific challenge related to health equality can be a bounded problem. The difference in colon cancer screening rates between black women and white women in a primary care clinic is a bounded problem. While this problem is an example of a health inequality, it has more specificity, so you can start to think of solutions—posting flyers in exam rooms, adding medical decision-making aids to the electronic health record, and assigning the responsibility of encouraging screening to a specific professional role, just for starters. It's not clear which of these solutions will work, but we've already come up with some promising ideas.

The most common reason advocacy fails is that the advocate is tackling an unbounded problem. Dream big, but concentrate your advocacy on a bounded problem.

Creating a Coalition

The next step in advocacy is to create a *coalition.* A coalition is a group of people with a shared interest, in this case, solving your bounded problem. For your coalition, you want to identify people who can speak to the problem, be they colleagues, patients and families, or others. Try to include as many diverse perspectives as feasible, but make sure that coalition members are committed to working on the problem. If someone can't or won't commit, consider how they might advise the process without being directly involved. You might need their help later. We will talk more about the importance of coalitions in the next chapter.

As you assemble your coalition, your understanding of the problem may change. The diversity of your coalition should influence how you see the problem. That's a good thing, so long as your problem stays bounded. As we did with group decision-making and navigating conflict, you need to have an open and free-flowing discussion around the problem to elicit different perspectives. This process will allow you to define a shared understanding of your specific problem, strengthen your coalition, and start to integrate diverse perspectives into your advocacy.

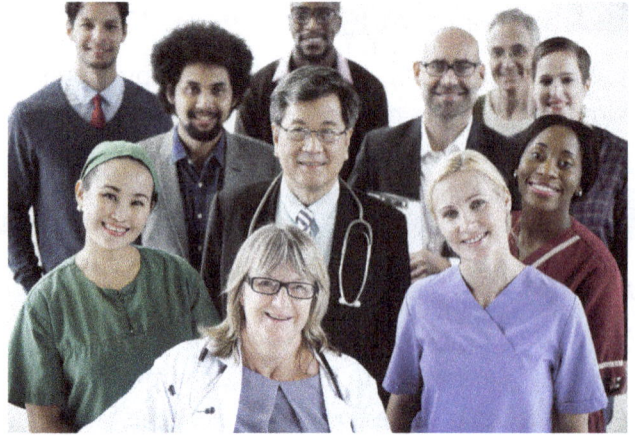

© Rawpixel.com/Shutterstock.com

Defining Solutions

Defining solutions shares a challenge with defining problems: we can be overly ambitious. Most of us want to change the world. But, as the Chinese proverb says, "A journey of a thousand miles begins with a single step." As the leader of the advocacy effort, it is your job to keep your coalition focused on the tangible first steps that will lead to sustainable change.

A useful way to do this is to think about solutions on two levels: short term and long term. While you need a long-term goal, you also need solutions that are small steps toward that larger vision. Smaller steps are simpler to describe and more pragmatic to implement. As a result, they are easier for leaders to endorse and increase your chance of successful advocacy. Small steps also help you learn about your problem and develop better solutions along the way to your long-term goal. The long-term goal is important for inspiration, but short-term solutions are the key to change and successful advocacy.

A good short-term solution has the following characteristics. It is:

- **Important:** It should feel like it will address an aspect of the problem in a way that matters to you and your colleagues.
- **Achievable:** It should be something you can actually do. As with a bounded problem, you want an initial solution that can be accomplished.
- **Momentum-building:** It should increase energy toward accomplishing your long-term goal. Consider at the outset how your solution, if successful, can spread or spur the next steps toward lasting change.

Your coalition may identify several possible short-term solutions. As you did when navigating conflict, you are trying to define the best of these possible solutions. When examining different solutions, there may be pros and cons in each of these three characteristics. Writing SMART goals for each

> **SMART Goals**
>
> SMART goals offer a good framework for defining short-term solutions. SMART is an acronym for:
> **S**pecific
> **M**easurable
> **A**chievable
> **R**elevant
> **T**ime-limited
>
> Defining a goal in this format forces us to focus our work and limit our aspirations, at least in the short term. SMART goals are typically written in a format like, "Four weeks from today, I will be able to run three miles without stopping to catch my breath." You can see the overlap between the characteristics of a good short-term solution and the ways that SMART goals further sharpen the boundaries around our solutions.

solution (see sidebar) can help clarify the merits of each approach. It can also be useful to think about how you can modify each solution to be more achievable or build more momentum. Your coalition may also need to seek out or incorporate additional perspectives. Making the best choice is important here—you might just get what you advocate for.

Advocating for Your Solution

Effective advocacy requires planning. While it may be tempting to go right to the top of a hierarchy and unveil your perfect solution, realize that your goal is to implement sustainable change. Working more systematically will increase your chance of having your solution both adopted and sustained. Let's look at some important strategies that can improve your likelihood of success.

Identify key decision-makers and key pressure-makers. Identifying key decision-makers may seem obvious, but sometimes it's unclear who makes decisions and how those decisions are made. Spend a few moments thinking through who is a key decision-maker for your problem. You don't want to miss anyone. In addition, think about why those decision-makers would be interested in your problem and inspired to implement your solution. Do some digging to see how those people have been involved with similar problems in the past.

Next, think about *pressure-makers*. Pressure-makers don't necessarily have formal power like decision-makers do, but they usually have relational power (see chapter 10). They know people; they have influence. They might be respected colleagues, community leaders, board members, or patients. Often, they have a track record of successful advocacy. Pressure-makers may come from within your coalition—it's a bonus to have influential colleagues already on your side—or your coalition members may be able to help identify and engage pressure-makers.

Pressure-makers are essential allies for advocacy (see figure 13.2). Rather than advocating alone to influence decision-makers, advocating with pressure-makers increases your chance of success. Diversity of pressure-makers is important; this allows you to represent different constituencies and advocate from different perspectives. Some decision-makers, especially ones who occupy intermediate positions in the organization's hierarchy, can also be enlisted as important pressure-makers with other decision-makers.

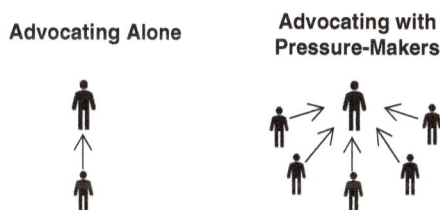

Figure 13.2 Advocating Alone Versus with Pressure-Makers. Source: Alan Dow.

Think about who to bring with you when you advocate to leaders. Sometimes, a colleague or patient might be a good advocacy partner. These people might have an essential perspective on the problem or the solution. But you don't want to overwhelm a leader with an office full of people. Most of us get apprehensive in front of a crowd, and the conversation may stall. You want the decision-maker's help and candid feedback. If you decide to bring someone with you to meet with a decision-maker, be sure that you understand each other's roles and are on the same page about the goals of the conversation.

Realize that you are starting a conversation. Decision-makers in healthcare are almost always moral, hard-working people who want to do the right thing for patients. However, one of their biggest challenges is having clarity about what is the right thing to do. Your job as an advocate is to bring them that clarity. To do that, you need to build a relationship so that they trust your assessment and your recommendations.

Realize that you are unlikely to get everything you want in your first meeting. Instead, start by outlining the problem and describing your work to date, including building your coalition and examining potential solutions. Highlight the solution that you recommend, but don't press for a decision. Instead, ask for their feedback and try to meet again in a couple of weeks. Most people need time to make decisions. And most leaders with lots of responsibilities will want some time to vet the problem and your solution with others. Your goal is to start a conversation and schedule a time to follow up.

Be specific and then adapt. Your description of the problem and the solution should be specific but not set in stone. While you don't need to present all the details, having them in writing—such as in a white paper—may help the leader review the conversation later. Realize that the decision-maker has a valuable perspective with considerations that you may not have contemplated. He or she may want to change your approach. Try to understand and clarify his or her underlying intentions (similar to the way you learned to resolve conflict in chapter 11) so that, as you adapt your solution now and in the future, you can integrate those rationales. Remember: the goal is to have another meeting and keep the conversation going.

Beyond the Decision-Maker

Even after you obtain the support of decision-makers, advocacy continues. Recall that formal power is only one of several types of power. You need to consider how people with expert power and relational power can help influence others to implement change. For example, key pressure-makers can be allies, or they can be barriers. How do you advocate with them for the change you want to see? In the final chapter, we will dive into this concept more deeply.

Advocacy in Interprofessional Practice

Let me emphasize several important concepts about advocating interprofessionally below and in the sidebar. Regardless of whether you are advocating for changes in organizational policy or additional resources for your area, the importance of professional diversity is clear. You want to make sure that you are representing the problem and its potential solutions accurately and thoughtfully. The best way to do that is to have a diversity of professional perspectives involved in your coalition.

> ### Athletic Trainers in IPE: A Step-by-Step Example of Advocacy
>
> Athletic training is one of the fastest-growing and most misunderstood professions. You may think of trainers as primarily working in sports-related settings, but they are increasingly employed by the military, performing arts organizations, and a variety of healthcare entities. Despite the growth of this profession in healthcare, athletic training is often overlooked as a health profession. Almost all of us need to learn more about athletic training. So, to address this problem and practice applying our advocacy principles, let's set the increased involvement of athletic trainers in interprofessional education (IPE) as an advocacy goal.
>
> But wait: increasing the involvement of athletic trainers in IPE is not a bounded problem. Yes, it's an important issue, but we need to start small. A bounded problem—and a better target for advocacy—is the lack of IPE experiences involving athletic training students at our (fictional) institution.

To tackle our bounded problem, we need to create our coalition. Who might be good coalition members? Faculty and students from the athletic training department and other professions seem to be obvious choices. We might also want to make sure we have some people with prior expertise in IPE and people who understand structures and hierarchies in universities. Perhaps you'd like to add other individuals as well.

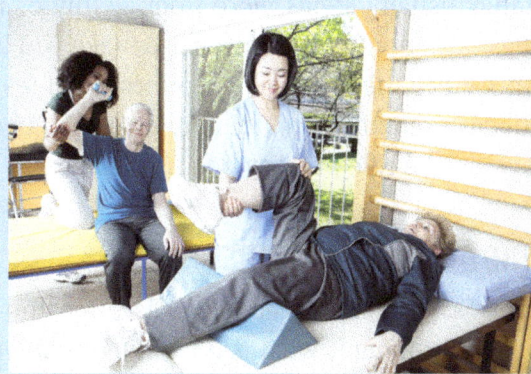

Then, our coalition needs to discuss potential solutions. Examples might be a classroom-based activity, a community service experience, or, my favorite, a trip to the sideline of some sporting event. Our coalition has to weigh the importance, practicality, and momentum-building of each solution and pick the best one as our short-term advocacy goal.

Finally, we are ready to advocate. We identify key decision-makers and pressure-makers. Our decision-makers are likely deans, program directors, and possibly other faculty. Our pressure-makers are faculty—some of whom may also be decision-makers—as well as students (who might be the most influential pressure-makers). We divide up these conversations based on prior relationships and start advocating. Game on!

In addition, think about the process of identifying and engaging pressure-makers. Key pressure-makers should come from many different areas of an organization or from society as a whole. Different members of your coalition may have more influence or access with certain pressure-makers. This influence may or may not follow professional lines: a chief medical officer who supervises doctors all day may only be receptive to advice from physicians. Alternatively, he or she may be accustomed to tuning out physician complaints, but, if a social worker shows up with a concern, that situation may be novel enough to spark a renewed engagement. Interprofessional pressure-making adds value.

Having an interprofessional approach also provides support as you work toward your goals. Working with interprofessional colleagues gives you more diverse feedback and better insight into how to integrate that feedback. Your coalition will also help you move past small failures and continue toward the larger goal of future success.

Finally, recognize the influence of interprofessional advocacy on the group itself. As an interprofessional group advocates, its members increase their internal and external relational power. They become a stronger and more effective team. Group members who are initially resistant or disengaged may become more active. It's not unusual for a solution's fiercest critic to become one of its strongest champions. As we advocate, we boost our collective strength, and that might be good for everyone's health.

Courage, Not Caution

If you are thinking about advocacy, you're likely already doing a great job in your role. You're competent enough to have the time and experience to think about the bigger picture, and you care enough to want to make change.

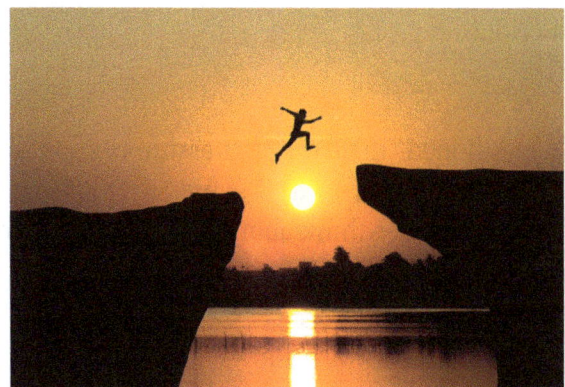

Be courageous. While advocacy is not without risk, this risk is often overstated. Yes, healthcare has politics, and some people will not be supportive, but this hesitancy usually stems more from apathy or inertia than disagreement. While you might get your feelings hurt, don't let a bruised ego make you lose sight of your goal. Advocacy is about helping your patients. Keep them—and your professional responsibility to them—in mind. Through advocacy, you will likely strengthen your relationships and become more influential. Someday, you might even find yourself in the role of a key decision-maker.

Application Questions

Defining a problem for advocacy is often the hardest step. Thinking about your current work or school environment, what is a bounded problem that you would like to see changed?

Who might be good members of a coalition to help define this problem, develop solutions, and advocate for change?

What might be an important, achievable, and momentum-building step toward this change? Articulate this step as a SMART goal.

Who might be key decision-makers to approach about this change?

Who might be key pressure-makers to help you advocate for this change?

Final Reflection Questions

As I noted, sometimes the fiercest critics of a change ultimately become the biggest advocates for that change. Why do you think that is? How might this observation influence how you think about a critic?

I mentioned that some pressure-makers are also decision-makers. What determines whether a decision-maker is also a pressure-maker? How might a decision-maker who is also a potential pressure-maker think about a problem and solution differently? How might you approach this type of decision-maker differently?

Compare and contrast internal advocacy (i.e., organizational change) with external advocacy (i.e., policy change). How might your coalition differ based on the type of advocacy you're engaged in? How might pressure-makers differ? How might you approach the process of advocacy differently?

Further Reading

Advocacy for Social Justice: A Global Action and Reflection Guide by David Cohen, Rosa de la Vega, and Gabrielle Watson (2001) describes advocacy efforts with case studies from around the world and provides several frameworks for how to advocate. Those frameworks were essential to developing this chapter.

Improving Healthcare Through Advocacy: A Guide for the Health and Helping Professions by Bruce Jansson (2011) is the best resource I found about advocating for individual patients. It's definitely worth reading if you have interest in this area.

Reporting of errors in healthcare has been recognized as a problem for over 20 years. The recent article, "Development of a Theoretical Framework of Factors Affecting Patient Safety Incident Reporting: A Theoretical Review of the Literature," by Stephanie Archer, Louise Hull, Tayana Soukup, Erik Mayer, Thanos Athanasiou, Nick Sevdalis, and Ara Darzi (2017), describes why error reporting is such a challenge and how we might do better.

CHAPTER 14

Building Trust and Improving Health

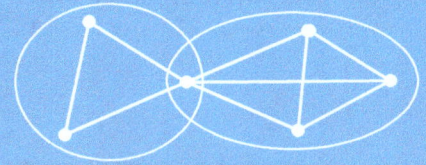

Throughout this book, we've looked at the mechanics of interprofessional practice and how you can best collaborate with others to care for your patients. One consistent theme has been the development of groups of practitioners into close-knit teams, through which we provide better, more shared care.

Now that we've reached the end of the book, it's time to look to the future and think about how our collaboration can drive change. Improving health is not just about your current patients and your current group of healthcare providers in your current setting. It's about the next planning-action cycle, the next resolved conflict, or the next consensus decision. As we saw in the last chapter, it's about combining our perspectives to create better ways of delivering care.

The purpose of this chapter—and this book overall—is to help you realize that future. By the end of this chapter, you will be able to:

▸ describe several frameworks for implementing change,
▸ identify the importance of relationships and coalition-building across traditional boundaries for effecting change, and
▸ explain how change can enhance collaboration and strengthen efforts to create future change.

Initial Reflection Questions

Think about a process of change that you have been involved in. It might be an organizational change related to work or school where you were directly involved in the process or a personal change where you wanted to improve something about yourself. How did you feel about the change? Did you prepare to make the change? If so, how?

What role did other individuals have in supporting the change process? How did the change process affect your relationships with them?

Did you successfully create change initially? Describe what helped and hindered your success.

Did the change stick, or did things revert back to their previous state? Describe what helped and what hindered when it came to maintaining the change.

Thinking About Change

Our goal in healthcare is positive change. At the level of the individual patient, we strive to make each patient healthier or, in the case of palliation, more comfortable. Across all of our patients, we hope to improve their overall health status while decreasing inequities and being a good steward of resources. For both our patients and our peers, we want the experience of interacting with each other to be better.

Our experiences provide us with expertise in our professional activities, the inner workings of the system, and the interface between patients and the healthcare system. Each of us is an expert in our setting and our professional role. We are uniquely positioned to think about how to make that practice environment better for ourselves, our colleagues, and our patients.

Our challenge is to convert our insights into visible change. Let's look at several overlapping models of change to help us think about that process. These models can apply to individuals or groups, but we will focus on the group and its impact on the organization. By presenting these models together, my hope is to build your capacity for thinking about and implementing change.

The Lewin Model of Change

Developed by Kurt Lewin, a social psychologist, the Lewin Model of Change has been applied to change in healthcare, especially in nursing. The model is a simple framework for thinking about change. We will use it as a foundation.

Let's depict change as the movement from an old practice to a better practice, though the model can also apply to other inputs and outputs of the change process. For now, think about the term "practice" broadly. This change could be creating a new norm as we discussed in group development, changing a specific behavior around patient care, or overhauling a major aspect of care.

In the Lewin Model (see figure 14.1), change happens because the driving forces for change are greater than the restraining forces against change. Your job, as a leader who wants to create change, is to enhance the driving forces and decrease the restraining forces. The process of creating this change has three steps: unfreeze, change, and refreeze.

Unfreezing means creating the conditions in which change can occur by leveraging the driving forces and limiting the restraining forces. Examples might include building a coalition and recruiting pressure-makers, as we discussed in the last chapter, or making sure that you have the resources for change to succeed. We'll discuss this unfreezing process in more depth in the next section. For now, just recognize that change requires preparation that is focused on the driving forces and restraining forces.

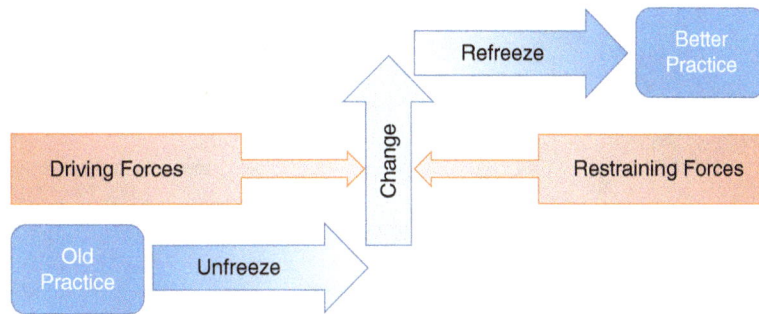

Figure 14.1 Lewin Model of Change Source: Alan Dow, based on the work of Kurt Lewin.

The *change* phase is when the new way of practice is implemented. This phase can feel unnatural because you are breaking norms. Though your target may be a change in professional activities and behaviors, change may also require new attitudes, knowledge, and skills. The group might go through a storming phase, and there can be conflict. Your work in the unfreezing phase seeks to lessen some of these challenges. However, because some people embrace change more easily than others, it is rare for change to go entirely smoothly. Expect to modify your approach during the change process as you see how your change impacts your setting.

The *refreeze* stage occurs when the change becomes engrained and is sustained. The new way of working becomes part of the culture—the way people behave when no one else is watching. The goal is for the change to evolve from an activity that requires conscious effort to the natural way that work is done.

The Kotter Model of Change

The Lewin Model can also be used as a framework for thinking about the stepwise Kotter Model of Change, created by John Kotter, a leadership professor. In contrast to the Lewin Model, Kotter provides a specific sequence of steps that are necessary for change. Five of these can be considered unfreezing steps, while three could be considered refreezing steps (see figure 14.2).

Kotter's first step is to *establish urgency*. Think of this as defining and emphasizing the driving forces for change. Why is change important? Why is it important now? As we discussed at the end of the chapter on negotiating, urgency is the cost of not deciding or not changing. You need to be able to articulate this cost to drive action in subsequent steps.

The second step is to *form a coalition*. As we've seen throughout this book, we are stronger when we work together as a diverse, collaborative group. By now, you are an expert in forming a group of collaborators. This step is simply a reminder to be deliberate and thoughtful about whom you include in your group.

Kotter named the third step *creating a vision*. Vision may be too broad a term for our purposes so creating a goal may be better. Remember our goal characteristics from the chapter on advocacy—important, achievable, and momentum-building.

The coalition is working to create and refine its vision or goal in the area of needed change. As with advocacy, our problem drives the creation of a shared solution. Your skills in identifying bounded

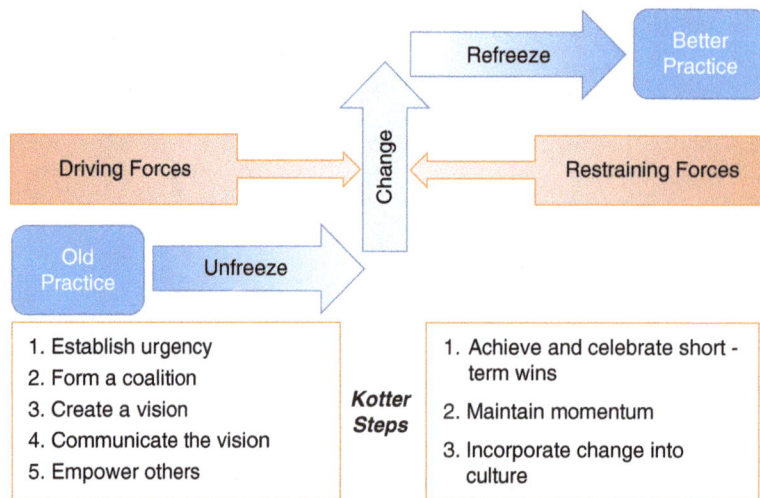

Figure 14.2 Lewin Model Integrated with Kotter Steps for Change Source: Alan Dow, based on the work on Kurt Lewin and John Kotter.

problems, creating consensus, and navigating conflict will be needed here as you establish what the change will actually look like.

The fourth and fifth steps are to *communicate the vision* and to *empower others*. Now that your coalition has a sense of what you want to do, you need to interact with those driving forces and restraining forces (such as decision-makers and pressure-makers) to make the change happen. Who do you need buy-in from so that change can happen—or who at least needs to get out of the way? Which of these people can you empower as additional members of your coalition to amplify your efforts? Think here about the different types of power: formal, expert, and relational. Who has the influence to improve your likelihood of success? You may need to practice your skills of followership here by sacrificing some of your role as a leader. Trust me, in the long run, everyone gets credit for successful change.

An important part of communicating the vision is developing simple messaging. Many worthwhile campaigns for change have succeeded or failed based on their ability to engage with people in their environment. Slogans work. We love catchy acronyms in healthcare. Think about how to brand your change so that you can engage everyone you need to. Your coalition can help create, test, and then disseminate your message.

Now we are ready to implement the change. If you have done a good job with unfreezing, using Kotter's first five steps, you will have generated a lot of enthusiasm around the change. However, that enthusiasm will wane quickly. Kotter helps us think about how to transition into refreezing to develop sustained change.

Kotter's sixth step is to *achieve and celebrate short-term wins*. With any change, you should seek out quick successes (an important, achievable, momentum-building solution). There may be early adopters who can be case studies for success, helping you advocate for expanding the change. Recognizing these successes reinforces the change and catalyzes others to join in the change movement. Take advantage of these opportunities to celebrate—who doesn't love a party?

The next-to-last step is to *maintain momentum*. This might be the most critical part of implementing change. At this point, the change is no longer the main area of focus. Everything you have done up to this point to enhance driving forces and decrease restraining forces, even when it has worked, may be losing impact. Yet somehow, you, your coalition, and your other colleagues must maintain the change. Your job is to keep everyone from slipping back into old behaviors as the new practice refreezes. This takes focus and ongoing effort.

Kotter's final step is to *incorporate change into culture*. As with the Lewin Model, the goal here is to make the change the way we naturally work. While formalizing the change through policies or modifications of the electronic health record are part of incorporating change, the informal and hidden ways in which the change becomes part of everyone's workflows and peer interactions are equally important. Think about the drivers of change from these different perspectives as you incorporate your change into your organization's culture.

The Transtheoretical Model of Change

Let's bring in one last model of change that may be familiar to you: the Transtheoretical Model. This model describes individual behavior changes like quitting smoking. As a model of change that can be applied clinically, it is worth comparing and contrasting with other models of change (see figure 14.3).

The Transtheoretical Model has five steps or stages of change. The first step is *precontemplation*. The underlying idea here is that a subconscious need for change begins to surface. The individual (or, for our purposes, the group or unit) has a need for change but has yet to become consciously aware of that need. A smoker who has no desire to quit despite the well-known hazards of smoking is in the precontemplation stage.

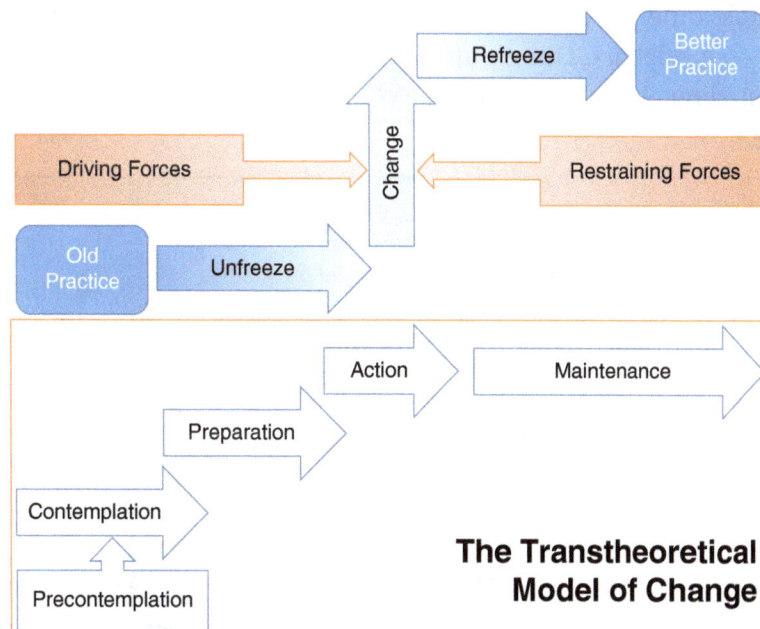

Figure 14.3 Comparing the Lewin and Transtheoretical Models Source: Alan Dow.

Contemplation is when the need for change becomes conscious. Now, a mental tug-of-war begins between the desire for change and the desire to maintain the old behavior. Applied to organizational change, urgency has begun to build, but there is not yet enough driving forces to move the change into Kotter's stages.

Next comes *preparation*. At this stage, we are unfreezing and moving into Kotter's first five steps. Like a smoker setting a quit date and marshaling family support for quitting, groups in the preparation stage are preparing to implement the change by making sure the necessary prerequisites are in order: coalition, vision, and empowerment.

Action is the stage in which we implement the change. For behavior change, this can be done quickly—stopping cold turkey—or through a prolonged phase of implementation like gradually tapering off a substance. Both for individuals and organizations, how to implement change in the action stage depends on what best fits the context.

Finally, *maintenance* is the phase of refreezing. How do you prevent slipping back into old behaviors and relapsing? This mirrors our process of maintaining momentum, and it's the most critical phase of change—making change stick is hard.

The Three Models of Change

The purpose of presenting these three models of change is to provide you with three overlapping perspectives. Several key themes are common to all the models, but each also has its own unique features. These features may help you anticipate challenges and get out of trouble as you implement change.

The first theme across the models is the need for preparation before implementing change. As we have seen across frameworks in this chapter and throughout this book, you need a diverse coalition. One of the most important abilities for creating change is the ability to be a boundary spanner: someone who can look across different professions or areas of work and identify who else has needed perspectives or abilities (see sidebar). Our group's impact depends on how well we can interact across all the diversity in our clinical environment.

(Sidebar) Boundary Spanners

Boundary spanners are people who overcome traditional boundaries to build relationships with people from another group. Examples of a group may be individuals from a profession, an area of work, or a circle of friends. For example, in figure 14.4, each dot represents a person; the lines are the connections between them. Those people are arranged into a peach group and a blue group. The individual indicated by the arrow is a boundary spanner, the person who connects two groups.

Boundary spanners are important for collaboration. They have unusual relational power through their connections with people across multiple groups. These connections make them more influential and provide them with a more diverse perspective.

Anyone can become a boundary spanner. It's as simple as cultivating relationships outside of your traditional groups. Consider how you can increase your capacity as a boundary spanner.

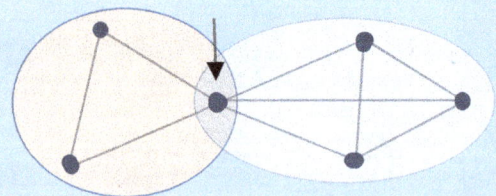

Figure 14.4 A Simple Social Network with an Arrow Indicating a Boundary Spanner, a Person Who Bridges Two Groups. Source: Alan Dow.

The second theme is that change is an ongoing process. In fact, each of these models depicts change as a straight line to success, which is an overly optimistic view. Change is an iterative process: as we try to change over and over, we get better at changing each time.

Think again about someone who wants to stop smoking. According to one study, the typical person who quits smoking tries 30 times before succeeding! Most of the times that smokers try to quit, they try new strategies to make their new efforts more successful. That's the iterative process in a nutshell—try to change, fail, make tweaks, try again, make more tweaks, and so on. Try changing your own behavior if you want to see how hard it is to change (see sidebar).

Learning About Change Through Personal Improvement

One way to understand how challenging change can be is to try to change yourself. This is a good exercise for understanding your patients' struggles with behavior changes and the challenges ahead of you as you work to make changes in your environment. This exercise is called a personal improvement plan, and it has five steps:

1. **Define a personal goal.** Make sure the goal you choose is something you care about and also something that's both measurable and time-limited. Frame it as a SMART goal as we talked about in the last chapter. Good examples of SMART personal goals are:
   "By four weeks from today, I want to run three miles without stopping."
   "By four weeks from today, I want to have written 10,000 words of my novel."
   "By four weeks from today, I want to be averaging eight hours of sleep per night over the previous two weeks."
2. **Identify some possible changes that could help you reach your goal.** Try to come up with three possible changes, and make sure these are concrete actions you can take. You might decide to do an activity when you first wake up. Or not do something after 10 p.m. Or do your new activity with a friend (this strategy works surprisingly well if you are both committed).
3. **Implement one change and track your progress.** Start with just one change and see how it goes. Make sure you have a system to track your progress relative to your goal.
4. **Iterate.** As you work toward your goal, you may find that some changes help while others don't. Some changes may be too challenging to implement. Or you may identify barriers to change that you hadn't considered. If you're not happy with your progress, try implementing a different change or tweaking a previous change.
5. **Reflect.** When you reach your deadline for your goal, think about how the change process went. Think about what changes helped you and why, as well as what barriers you encountered and how you overcame them (or didn't).

The purpose of this exercise is not strictly to change yourself; it's to learn about the process of implementing change and make you a wiser practitioner as a result.

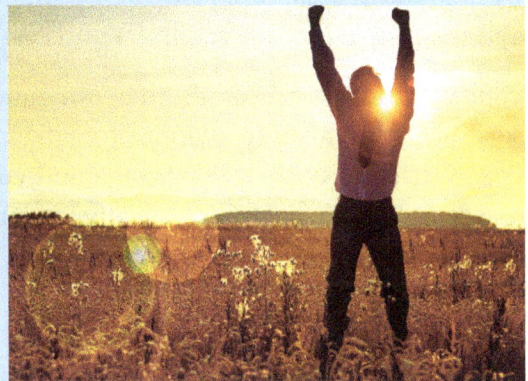

© conrado/Shutterstock.com

Several other models for change use the ongoing process of change to make improvements in quality. PDSA (Plan-Do-Study-Act) is the most widely used of these quality-improvement models. In PDSA, you "plan" a change, "do" it (implement an action), "study" the effects, and "act" on your results to make tweaks and plan a new change, restarting the process. A successful quality-improvement project may go through many PDSA cycles as the intervention gets better and better. Think of change as a continual, iterative process.

Finally, the last theme across the models is the need to maintain the end state of change—through refreezing, incorporating the change into culture, and maintenance. In each of the models, this final step does not represent a conclusion. Rather, the process of solidifying change continues over time. Individuals or a system can revert back to an earlier state even long after change is implemented. We have to focus on sustainability.

To reach sustainability, the Kotter Model focuses on the importance of small wins and maintaining momentum, while the Transtheoretical Model emphasizes the maintenance phase. The key point is that change is an ongoing process that involves repeated failure. We need to learn from failure and be flexible about altering course in response to it. A strengths-based model (chapter 12) can help here. The problem that's driving the change isn't going away, so we need to help our patients and our colleagues be resilient as they refreeze into a new way of doing things.

Avoiding Failure

The most common reason for a failure to change is that the attempted change is too big. If you smoke to manage your stress, it's a bad idea to try to quit smoking during a stressful holiday season. Likewise, if you're trying to implement some significant organizational change, make sure your workplace is ready for it. As we discussed in the advocacy chapter, you need to identify bounded problems with bounded solutions. And you need to do your preparation in advance so that your environment and the people in it are set up for success.

Your coalition is essential. Someone may get frustrated by the difficulty of the unfreezing process. You may need to alter your change or shrink your first effort. If you get to the point where you've tried to implement change and your efforts keep failing, don't give up. Take a step back, reassemble your coalition, and figure out what went wrong so you can decide how to proceed differently.

Trust, Change, and Improving Health

There's another reason to try to change the way that we care for people. Yes, we ultimately want to improve people's health, and changing the system is one way to try to do that. But the process of change has another effect—one that spills over onto us and the people we work with. Striving for change makes us articulate what we believe in, imagine what a better future might look like, and strategize ways to come together around those ideals.

In her excellent writing about what she calls relational coordination, Jody Hoffer Gittell, a management professor, describes how some coordination or networking groups perform better than others. She identifies three important factors influencing that difference: the structures that support the groups, the processes that shape how group members interact, and the strength of the relationships among group members. Your change efforts might advocate for new group structures and processes. Those changes are important. But it's equally important to recognize how change itself brings us together. Through working on change, we get the added benefit of strengthening our relationships.

I previously described leadership as a team, rather than individual, concept, in that leadership grows as our group becomes more of a team. Capacity for change is similar. By moving through the change process, we increase our team's capacity for change. We develop trust and a sense of shared purpose with our colleagues. Our groups become more resilient as we also become more effective.

So, go out and change the world. Your patients are counting on you.

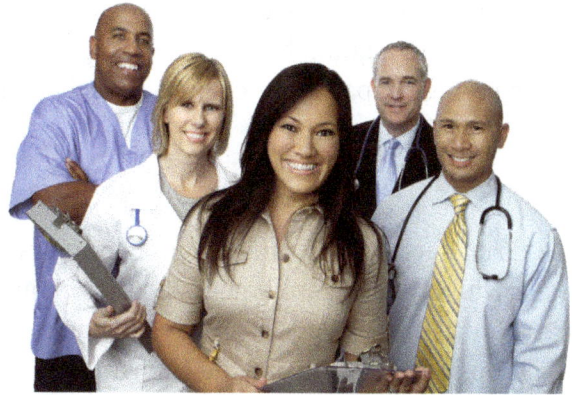

Application Questions

Identify a change that you would like to make in your life.

What are the driving forces or reasons to make this change?

What are the restraining forces or reasons not to make this change?

Who are the key people—your coalition—who could help you make this change? How could you engage them to support you as you make this change?

Who could hamper your efforts at change? Are these people similar to the members of your coalition, or are they different? How can you engage these people to prevent them from hampering your change?

What are some short-term wins or early accomplishments that will signify your success at implementing this change?

What are some of the challenges to maintain this change? What are some approaches that you could use to help you overcome these challenges?

Final Reflection Questions

Think about the potential for boundary spanning in your current or future career. In that setting, what are some of the other groups that affect your work? How can you span the boundaries between these groups and your existing groups? What strategies might you use to span those boundaries? How might spanning boundaries benefit you, the individuals in the other groups, and your patients?

I described the capacity for change as something that groups have as a collective quality. What are the benefits of a group having a high capacity for change? What might be some downsides of a group having a high capacity for change, especially at the broader system level?

We discussed urgency and vision as important precursors for change. What is a healthcare-related issue where you feel an urgent need for change? What would your vision be for that change? What are the driving forces for change and the restraining forces against change? Who might be in your coalition to help you make the change?

Further Reading

John Kotter's most famous book is *Leading Change: An Action Plan From the World's Foremost Expert on Business Leadership* (1988). In it, he describes his model and its implications. He also has written about the importance of urgency for change; see his book *Our Iceberg Is Melting: Changing and Succeeding Under Any Conditions* (2006) for more on that topic.

Several authors have written about boundary spanners in healthcare. If you want to read more, a good place to start is the article "Bridges, Brokers and Boundary Spanners in Collaborative Networks: A Systematic Review," by Janet Long, Frances Cunningham, and Jeffrey Braithwaite in *BMC Health Services Research* (2013).

Jody Hoffer Gittell has a number of excellent books on group performance and how to improve it. Her best-known book, *The Southwest Airlines Way: Using the Power of Relationships to Achieve High Performance* (2002), looked at how Southwest Airlines dominated the competition by supporting dispersed groups to enable them to function more like teams. She then applied those same principles to healthcare in the book *High Performance Healthcare: Using the Power of Relationships to Achieve Quality, Efficiency and Resilience* (2009). Her most recent book, *Transforming Relationships for High Performance: The Power of Relational Coordination* (2016), is also excellent; it expands on her healthcare work with case studies from several healthcare organizations.

INDEX

Speech therapist, 92
Storming, 70–71
Stroke, speech-language pathologist and, 32
Subacute nursing facility (SNF), 80–81

T

Task conflict, 112–113
Team, mature form of group as, 68. *See also* Groups
Teamwork
    challenges to, 50
    defined, 50
    fixing problems in healthcare, 51
    group process and, 78
360-degree feedback, 124
Transtheoretical Model of Change
    action, 148
    contemplation, 148
    maintenance, 148
    precontemplation, 147
    preparation, 148
Trust building and health improvement
    application questions, 151
    change
        Kotter Model of, 145–147
        Lewin Model of, 144–145
        purpose of models of, 148–150
        reason for failure to, 150
        Transtheoretical Model of, 147–148

reflection questions
    final, 151–152
    initial, 143–144
Tuckman's stages of group development, 68.
    See also specific stages

U

Unbounded problems, 135
Urgency to make decision, 95

V

Vaccination, 59

W

Work
    application questions, 45
    chaotic, 45
    and collaboration, integrating, 52–53
    complex, 44–45
    complicated, 43–44
    reflection questions
        final, 46
        initial, 41
    simple, 42–43
Workaround, 90–91
Work team, 68